Treatment of Suicidal Patients in Managed Care

Treatment of Suicidal Patients in Managed Care

Edited by

James M. Ellison, M.D., M.P.H.

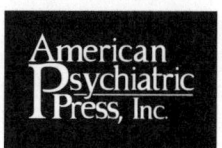

Washington, DC
London, England

Note: The authors have worked to ensure that all information in this book concerning drug dosages, schedules, and routes of administration is accurate as of the time of publication and consistent with standards set by the U.S. Food and Drug Administration and the general medical community. As medical research and practice advance, however, therapeutic standards may change. For this reason and because human and mechanical errors sometimes occur, we recommend that readers follow the advice of a physician who is directly involved in their care or the care of a member of their family.

Books published by the American Psychiatric Press, Inc., represent the views and opinions of the individual authors and do not necessarily represent the policies and opinions of the Press or the American Psychiatric Association.

Copyright © 2001 American Psychiatric Press, Inc.
ALL RIGHTS RESERVED
Manufactured in the United States of America on acid-free paper

04 03 02 01   4 3 2 1
First Edition

American Psychiatric Press, Inc.
1400 K Street, N.W.
Washington, DC 20005
www.appi.org

Library of Congress Cataloging-in-Publication Data
Treatment of suicidal patients in managed care /   edited by James M. Ellison.—1st ed.
    p. ; cm.
Includes bibliographical references and index.
ISBN 0-88048-828-X (alk. paper)
    1. Suicide—Prevention. 2. Suicidal behavior—Treatment. 3. Managed care plans (Medical care). 4. Managed care plans (Medical care)—Patients—Care. I. Ellison, James M., 1952–
    [DNLM: 1. Suicide—psychology. 2. Managed Care Programs. 3. Suicide—prevention & control. WM 165 T784 2001]
RC569 .T736 2001
616.85'8445—dc21
                                                         00-056946

British Library Cataloguing in Publication Data
A CIP record

```
616.89 T784e



Treatment of suicidal
   patients in managed care
```

Contents

Contributors... vii

Acknowledgments ix

Foreword xi
    James Harburger, M.D.

CHAPTER 1

Treating Suicidal Patients in the Managed Care Environment.......... 1
    John T. Maltsberger, M.D.

CHAPTER 2

Managed Crisis Care for Suicidal Patients........................ 15
    Judith Feldman, M.D.
    Linda Finguerra, R.N., C.S.

CHAPTER 3

Managed Care, Brief Hospitalization, and Alternatives to
Hospitalization in the Care of Suicidal Patients................... 39
    Patricia A. Harney, Ph.D.

CHAPTER 4

Suicidal Adolescents in Managed Care........................... 59
    Alan Lipschitz, M.D.

CHAPTER 5

Suicide in the Elderly 85
    Ashok Bharucha, M.D.

CHAPTER 6

Substance Abuse and Suicidal Behavior in Managed Care........... 111
    Richard Caplan, M.S.W., M.P.H.

CHAPTER 7

Psychiatric Pharmacotherapy, Suicide, and Managed Care 131
James M. Ellison, M.D., M.P.H.

CHAPTER 8

Risk Management Issues for Clinicians Who Treat
Suicidal Patients in Managed Systems. 153
Catherine Keyes, J.D.

CHAPTER 9

In the Aftermath of Suicide: Needs and Interventions 173
Steve Stelovich, M.D.

APPENDIX A

The Formulation of Suicide Risk 189
John T. Maltsberger, M.D.

APPENDIX B

Getting More of What Is Needed From Your
Patient's Managed Care Organization 197
James M. Ellison, M.D., M.P.H.

Index 203

CONTRIBUTORS

Ashok Bharucha, M.D., is an assistant professor of psychiatry at University of Pittsburgh School of Medicine, Pittsburgh, Pennsylvania.

Richard Caplan, M.S.W., M.P.H., is a faculty member of the Zinberg School for Studies in the Addictions at Harvard Medical School, and former manager of Substance Abuse Services for Harvard Vanguard Medical Associates in Boston, Massachusetts. He is currently on the adjunct faculty of Boston University School of Social Work and in private practice in Cambridge, Massachusetts.

James M. Ellison, M.D., M.P.H., is an associate clinical professor in psychiatry at Harvard Medical School, a consultant to The Cambridge Hospital Psychiatry Department, and clinical director of ambulatory services and of geriatric psychiatry at McLean Hospital in Belmont, Massachusetts. He is also a past president of the board of the Northeast Affiliate of the American Foundation for Suicide Prevention.

Judith Feldman, M.D., is an assistant clinical professor of psychiatry at Harvard Medical School and was chief of Central Mental Health Programs at Harvard Vanguard Medical Associates in Boston, Massachusetts.

Linda Finguerra, R.N., C.S., is a psychiatric nurse clinical specialist and nurse clinician. She is also the coordinator of the Intensive Dialectical Behavior Therapy Program at Harvard Vanguard Medical Associates in Boston, Massachusetts.

James Harburger, M.D., is an Instructor in Psychiatry at Harvard Medical School and former Director of Mental Health Services at Harvard Vanguard Medical Associates in Boston, Massachusetts.

Patricia A. Harney, Ph.D., was formerly on staff at Boston Regional Medical Center, where she worked with the Managed Care Team. She is a clinical instructor in psychology at The Cambridge Hospital, Harvard Medical School, and a clinical psychologist in private practice in Cambridge, Massachusetts.

Catherine Keyes, J.D., is an attorney and a loss prevention staff consultant at the Risk Management Foundation of the Harvard Medical Institutions in Cambridge, Massachusetts. She is president of the Massachusetts Society of Healthcare Risk Management.

Alan Lipschitz, M.D., is Medical Director, CNS, at Wyeth-Ayerst Pharmaceuticals, Philadelphia, Pennsylvania.

John T. Maltsberger, M.D., is an associate clinical professor of psychiatry at Harvard Medical School; an attending psychiatrist at McLean Hospital in Belmont, Massachusetts; and a clinical associate in psychiatry at Massachusetts General Hospital in Boston.

Steve Stelovich, M.D., is an instructor in psychiatry at Harvard Medical School and medical director of the Arbour Fuller Hospital in Attleboro, Massachusetts.

ACKNOWLEDGMENTS

In October 1996, the contributors to this book joined together to explore the multifaceted and evolving relationships between new health care delivery systems and the care of suicidal patients. The American Foundation for Suicide Prevention and Harvard Pilgrim Health Care assisted us in organizing the conference on which this book in part is based, entitled "Providing Effective Managed Care for the Suicidal Patient," and the generous unrestricted support of Abbott Laboratories, Eli Lilly and Company, Pfizer, Searle, SmithKline Beecham, Solvay Pharmaceuticals, Inc., and Wyeth-Ayerst Laboratories helped us bring our ideas to the podium.

Our sense of the importance of this discussion was so greatly reinforced by the responsiveness of our audience that we determined to prepare the present collection of essays. Our hope is that this book will prove useful to clinicians who treat suicidal patients within managed care programs or under managed care insurances, administrators developing procedures to aid suicidal patients, and managed care planners seeking to improve the quality of care delivered to these complex individuals.

The collaborative process by which this book was produced brought together clinicians from private practice and managed settings, authorities on suicide and related topics, and managed care administrators engaged in the continuing process of program development and outcome measurement. Each provides a unique perspective on the relationship between suicide and managed care, and to each I would like to express my gratitude for sharing valuable insights into the ways in which we can improve our clinical effectiveness. To my wife, Patricia, who shared her dual expertise in managed care and private practice treatment, I owe special gratitude. She not only contributed a chapter but also served as the first reader of many others' chapter drafts. Her helpful comments prevented several of us from straying too far afield. More importantly, she sacrificed my companionship at many hours in order to smooth the path to this book's completion in time for us to share, relatively unencumbered, in the miraculous birth of our son Daniel, whom we both wish to welcome into this rapidly changing, remarkable world.

FOREWORD

The rapid recent growth of managed health care, followed by the even more rapid proliferation of managed behavioral health care organizations (MBHCOs), has had a dramatic and far-reaching impact on the practice of psychiatry and the related mental health professions, hospitals, and community based programs. Clinicians have experienced an assault on the autonomy of their decision making, the confidentiality of the treatment process, and anticipated levels of reimbursement for their work. The trends away from long-term to short-term treatment, from individual to group therapy, from hospital to day treatment, and from psychotherapy to pharmacotherapy reflect a change process with a surprisingly fast pace. Compounding the distress accompanying these shifts in the clinical practice culture has been the arrival of the utilization reviewer: a person empowered to intrude into the treatment relationship, to approve or deny coverage of care, to decide whose hospitalization will be paid for and for how long, and to decide how many outpatient visits will be reimbursed, for what kind of therapy, and by which clinician. Were this intrusive authority not sufficiently disconcerting, these reviewers also often require the clinician to fill out complex forms, differing from one MBHCO to another, and these must be completed and submitted to allow for discussions or arguments to take place regarding authorizations for continued care, for diagnostic studies such as neuropsychological testing, or for additional consultations.

As some individual clinicians find employment in staff model health maintenance organizations or networks, including even some community mental health programs, they encounter "capitation arrangements," and their discussions about utilization management shift from interactions with external reviewers to feedback from colleagues. The concept of *population based* requires us to scrutinize what services a patient should receive and at what cost to the patient, the insurer, and society. Discussion about how most expeditiously and least expensively to achieve desired therapeutic goals must be addressed. What level and intensity of care are required? What is the evidence to support the use of more expensive treatments, when less costly but equally effective alternatives exist? In contrast to the earlier fee-for-service culture where we grew concerned about the possibility that excessive amounts of care were provided to generate greater clinician and hospital incomes, we now discuss our ethical concerns about the danger of profits and bonuses being tied to withholding of care.

In this new mix of forces has also been a sentiment of entitlement to services among some patients, a feeling they have *prepaid* for them. At the same time, the MBHCOs are responding to these requests for psychotherapy by using the criteria of medical necessity to guide decisions about authorization. As the controversy intensifies over what conditions and level of distress meet the test of medical necessity, patients, clinicians, and policymakers have all contributed their views.

It is in the midst of these changes and conflicts that our suicidal patients continue to present for evaluation and treatment. We know that suicide remains an all too common cause of death, and we wish to see our patients well and safely served. Suicide remains one of the 10 leading causes of death in the United States and the third leading cause of death in adolescents, accounting for 30,000 deaths annually in this country. And while suicide may seem the only feasible course of action to a tormented, depressed, or psychotic patient, we clinicians know that it is one of the more preventable forms of death and that many survivors of suicide attempts are able to find alternative ways to cope with the stresses that elicited self-destructive behavior. It is at the intersection of managed care systems and psychiatric evaluation and treatment of our most vulnerable and suicidal patients that this book seeks to provide guidance and perspective.

When a MBHCO works well, the evaluation and referral process considers what is the best treatment match to help this patient most quickly achieve symptomatic relief and behavior change. It asks should this patient see a male or female therapist? Would he or she be better treated individually, as part of a couple or family, in a group alone, or in combination? Is a psychodynamic or cognitive-behavioral modality most likely to be helpful? Is the patient's presentation likely to be dealt with in a general practice or to require consultation and care with a subspecialist? Is pharmacotherapy likely to be central, adjunctive, or unneeded? Can this treatment take place in an office setting, or does it require a hospital, partial hospital, or acute residential program? Do the patient, clinician, and reviewer have a shared understanding about the treatment plan, insurance coverage, authorization process, and the need and timing of treatment reviews and reauthorization discussions.

A MBHCO may underserve a patient, failing to provide the care that is needed, but this is often a reflection of misunderstandings, inadequate communication, inflexibility, or poor resolution of disagreements. Harried clinicians, feeling that they have too little time for patients and too many procedural demands required to obtain authorizations for additional clinical services, become increasingly frustrated. In this context, therapists can end up joining with their patients in complaining about the MBHCO, treatment decisions may be less well thought out, and dreaded outcomes may occur. In those circumstances there are no happy participants. Clinicians, hospitals, MBHCOs, and their legal and risk management departments approach such occurrences with understandable trepidation.

In the first chapter of this book, John T. Maltsberger explores the risks to suicidal patients when MBHCOs intrude into clinical decision making by refusing admissions and pushing for early discharges. Evaluations may be constrained, treatments may not yet be fully effective at the time of discharge, and the hospital and program structure needed for safe recovery may be denied or withdrawn too soon. Dr. Maltsberger emphasizes—and this cannot be stressed too emphatically—that an initial thorough assessment of a patient and formulation are made all the more crucial when treatment is constrained to a shortened interval by managed care.

In the second chapter, Judith Feldman and Linda Finguerra explore the provision of crisis assessments and care for suicidal patients in a managed care practice. They underscore the importance of easily available, barrier-free access to assessments and care for such patients to ascertain the danger of self-harm and to clarify the appropriate level and locus of treatment required. They then review the difficult problem inherent in assessing the repeatedly self-harming patient with personality disorder. These authors outline an approach to helping the suicidal patient in crisis by making use of cognitive-behavioral strategies and the techniques described by Marsha Linehan, under the rubric of dialectic behavior therapy (DBT), including the development of new coping strategies, contingency planning, behavioral analysis, and the search for available supports.

In Chapter 3, Patricia A. Harney reviews the role of brief hospitalization and alternative programs such as acute residential care and day hospitals in treating suicidal patients. She reminds us of the value of emergency rooms and crisis services as consultants to patients, families, and therapists who are all fearful of a lethal outcome. She underscores the importance at such times for the ambulatory therapist of knowing whom to call in the managed care system to access crisis assessments and evaluations for hospital levels of care. Her discussion of partial hospital and acute residential care stresses the value of these less regressive options for patients who can voluntarily agree to care at such treatment sites and who have fewer needs for medical supervision or for the secure environment of a locked hospital ward.

In Chapter 4, Alan Lipschitz draws our attention to the pressing public health concern of adolescent suicide. He notes concern that brief inpatient stays create intense pressures for the treatment staff to complete an evaluation, including family assessment and involvement in treatment planning. He observes that when admissions are too short, distressing, and costly, readmissions may follow. Here again, the value of multiple levels of care, including home treatment and long-term residential care, is stressed. Lastly, he notes with concern the disruption to the care process that can occur when a family's insurance changes and a child's therapist is not on the new carrier's provider panel.

In Chapter 5, Ashok Bharucha addresses suicide risks in the elderly. Suicide rates increase with age. With the aging of our population and the increasing recruitment of seniors into managed care plans, there is a renewed interest in training primary care physicians in the diagnosis and treatment of depression. This is particularly important in light of studies that have shown that such physicians often underdiagnose and undertreat depression and that they may be uncomfortable asking questions about suicidal ideation and intention. This chapter contains a wonderful menu of preventative interventions to keep the elderly active, socially well supported, and depression free.

In Chapter 6, Richard I. Caplan explores the relationship between substance abuse and suicide. He notes both the high rate of suicide attempts in substance abusers and the high percentage of people who attempt suicide while intoxicated. He suggests that MBHCOs are advantageously structured to screen populations for both substance abuse and depression in the context of medical, pediatric, and obstetrical visits. He then addresses the familiar and vexing problem of suicide assessments of intoxicated alcoholic individuals and drug-addicted individuals and highlights the need to detain patients for reevaluation until they are sober. He goes on to describe a broad spectrum of services that are helpful in treating substance abusers. This is followed by a discussion of the role of case managers in providing continuity of care in a disorder known to be chronic and relapsing. We are reminded that effective treatment of substance abuse disorders should not only reduce the likelihood of suicidal outcomes but also improve patients' general state of health and well-being and decrease their overall health care costs.

In Chapter 7, James M. Ellison reviews the pharmacotherapy of depression and suicidality and the potential supports and constraints of MBHCOs. Medication and electroconvulsive therapy (ECT) have come to play a crucial role in reducing suicidal mortality. The role of each class of medication is reviewed as well as their target symptoms and disorders. The risks, benefits, and issues surrounding who does the prescribing and their level of expertise are thoughtfully explored. This is increasingly relevant, because in many managed care settings primary care physicians have begun to play a major role in treating uncomplicated unipolar depression. Dr. Ellison also raises concerns about the adequacy of visit lengths and frequency authorized by MBHCOs, the large multimonth prescriptions patients receive to reduce MBHCO costs and patients' copayments, the use of restrictive formularies, and the adequacy of outreach and follow-up for patients who miss appointments.

In Chapter 8, Catherine Keyes reviews risk management considerations associated with the treatment of suicidal patients in managed care settings. Areas of potential concern include ensuring diagnostic accuracy, choosing the appropriate treatment, and monitoring shifting levels of risks. Other important decision points include when to use and to discontinue "specials" in the hospital, the use of restraints, safety of patient rooms, adequacy of documentation of care, and arrangement for follow-up after discharge. Communication and careful passing of the baton of responsibility are also critical care junctures. Lastly, she reminds us that since managed care companies can be perceived as profiting from withholding care, documenting the reasons for treatment decisions is of extreme importance.

In Chapter 9, Steve Stelovich provides a model for managing the aftermath of a suicide. He offers an elegant road map for dealing with the treating clinicians, bereaved family and friends, other affected patients on a hospital unit or in a group, and the medical care system supporting the treatment. He then walks the reader through consideration of four processes affecting each of these groups: 1) anticipation of such an event, 2) announcing or sharing the news of a suicide, 3) assessing those impacted, and 4) seeing what can be learned from reviewing the patient's treatment.

In a helpful and concise first appendix, Dr. Maltsberger returns to offer a model for assessing suicidal risk. He reminds us to review how the patient managed past times of stress, to evaluate how vulnerable is the patient to life-threatening affect, how available are sustaining resources, how present and malevolent are fantasies about death, and, lastly, how compromised is the patient's capacity to reality test. Dr. Ellison provides an additional brief appendix with concrete tips for the clinician who must understand a patient's benefits and advocate for further services with an MBHCO.

In these times of rapid change in the structure of mental health service delivery systems, this book describes how managed mental health may improve or impede the care of suicidal patients. It highlights the risks, constraints, and supports patients and therapists may uncover as they interact with MBHCOs. The book provides timely advice and guidance. I hope it will be one that you will want to keep at hand and refer to often, since it contains the collected experience and wisdom of many thoughtful colleagues.

James Harburger, M.D.

CHAPTER 1

Treating Suicidal Patients in the Managed Care Environment

John T. Maltsberger, M.D.

The incursion of "managed care" into American medicine during the past 15 years has profoundly disrupted the care of psychiatric and other patients. The thrusting of ever greater numbers of patients into outpatient settings has been proposed as one of the factors responsible for the dramatic 2.57-fold increase in the number of deaths from accidental poisonings and medication errors in the United States between 1983 and 1993 (Phillips et al. 1998a), mediated perhaps through the increased use of more powerful drugs on an outpatient basis, an increased average number of doses prescribed per prescription (see also Chapter 7, this volume, for discussion of this issue), and an increase in the number of illnesses considered treatable on an outpatient basis (Manasse 1998). We read reports of suicides that seem to follow when managed care reviewers compel hospital discharge through premature termination of insurance benefits (Schouten 1993; Sharfstein 1989; Westermeyer 1991). Furthermore, managed care insurers commonly refuse to pay for partial hospital programs and thereby deprive patients of the structure clinicians feel they need for safe recovery (Lewin 1990).

Our patients and their caregivers suffer through a chaotic era. The limited time possible for inpatient workups and treatment, the decimation of inpatient staff, and the rapid increase in rates of admission and discharge demand greater familiarity with the principles of assessment and management, and increased efficiency in their use, if our patients' are to be treated as safely and intelligently as the times permit.

Constraints of space preclude a detailed discussion of the principles of suicide risk assessment, but the reader may find the first appendix (see Appendix A) at the back of this book helpful. The fullest recent treatment of this subject is that of Maris and colleagues (1992).

Diagnosis

Though diagnosis alone is never sufficient to settle questions of management and treatment, at least it orients the busy clinician to some extent. Because the majority of suicides occur in the context of a major mental illness, we may assert the general rule that ameliorating the suffering of persons with these illnesses can be expected to diminish the risk of suicide. ("Major mental illness" refers here to the so-called Axis I disorders as set forth in DSM-IV [American Psychiatric Association 1994] and most recently in its text revision, DSM-IV-TR [American Psychiatric Association 2000].) Correct diagnosis and the treatment appropriate for it is clearly a matter of early priority.

Depressive Illness

All the principal investigations of diagnosis following suicide indicate that major depressive illness is the most common and most highly associated diagnosis. Barraclough and colleagues (1974) reported this disorder in 74% of deaths from suicide, Dorpat and Ripley (1960) in 28%, and Robins and coworkers (1959) in 47%. In my opinion, it is virtually always present in schizophrenic and alcoholic individuals who commit suicide and in suicidal patients with borderline and other personality disorders.

Evidence is accumulating that the kind of depression that invites suicide is comparatively more specialized than that defined by DSM-IV's broad embrace. That is to say, some of the depressive indicia listed in that book appear to be more deadly than others.

Shneidman has emphasized the importance of mental suffering in driving suicide, venturing to call it "psychache"; in fact, he says that psychache causes suicide (Shneidman 1993). Though anguish (suffering in the mind, psychache, psychic anxiety, mental agony, horror, terror) is commonplace in depression, it is not listed with the discrete specificity it deserves among the DSM-IV diagnostic criteria for that disorder. If it is among the criteria at all, it is lost in the mists of criterion A1, which refers to "depressed mood" as though what constituted such an affective experience were fairly evident (American Psychiatric Association 1994, pp. 320–321). It behooves examiners to look closely into the level of *mental anguish* their patients experience.

Dictionaries define anguish as extreme pain, distress, or anxiety (see, e.g., Mish 1983). Shneidman (1993) defines psychache, which I take for a synonym for mental anguish, as follows:

> *Psychache* refers to the hurt, anguish, soreness, aching, psychological pain in the psyche, the mind. It is intrinsically psychological—the pain of excessively felt shame, or guilt, or humiliation, or loneliness, or fear, or angst, or dread. . . . When it occurs, its reality is introspectively undeniable. (p. 51)

Historically, it has been assumed that intense mental suffering of the anxious, agitated kind is part of classical depression; Kraepelin recognized it for a danger signal long ago (Kraepelin 1921, pp. 39, 95; see Maltsberger 1986). More recently, there has been a tendency to split anxiety states off from depression and to treat them as a separate diagnostic group, as in DSM-IV. Whether we think of patients' anxiety as being comorbid with a depressive disorder (the contemporary trend) or whether we understand the experience of painful psychic anxiety to belong, part and parcel, to the dysphoria of major depression, clinically it is a bad sign.

Fawcett (1997) has brought home how important it is to seek out signs of anxiety in depression, emphasizing the importance of anguish in suicide risk assessment. In the first place, the presence of intense anxiety is closely correlated with the severity of the overall depressive experience. The severity of psychic anxiety and the presence of panic attacks are significantly correlated with suicide within the first year of follow-up. Furthermore, preliminary review (a "nonblinded" analysis) of some 75 inpatient suicide records showed clear evidence of severe anxiety-agitation in 78% of the cases in the week before suicide. Fawcett properly emphasizes that severe anxiety once detected must be treated to reduce the risk of suicide.

Examiners should not assume they can correctly estimate the level of mental suffering by inferring from a patient's general appearance and behavior. Specific direct inquiry is in order.

Case Example

> A 25-year-old graduate student was admitted to the hospital in a severely retarded state. He slumped in his chair, moved about very little, and answered questions in monosyllables. There was no outward indication of

agitation. Nevertheless, the patient was asked to rate his level of mental anguish from 0 to 5, where 0 would indicate no mental pain, and 5, such agony that he would have to dash screaming down the corridor or kill himself to escape it. After a long pause, he replied, "Four and a half." The next day, still in a retarded state, he jumped in front of a delivery van as he was escorted to the cafeteria, only narrowly escaping injury.

Clinical experience indicates that a substantial degree of self-hate,[1] when coupled with moderate to severe anguish, increases the risk of death by suicide. In my opinion, the patient who evinces significant degrees of anguish, self-hate, and hopelessness all at the same time is suicidal, even if he denies suicide on direct inquiry. While Fawcett and colleagues (1990) did not find that *hopelessness* at the index admission of a large series of affective disorder patients predicted suicide in the first year of follow-up, it makes good clinical sense to regard patients who display anguish, self-hate, and hopelessness at the same time with great concern.

Plainly, we need to know more than we do about which affective experiences drive patients to suicide. Common sense suggests that mental anguish, the most painful aspect of depressive dysphoria, is likely to promote suicide more than feeling numb, for instance. Surprisingly little empirical work has been done to break down and characterize the dysphoria of major depression, though Zanarini and colleagues (1998) have begun to sort out the various components of dysphoria as experienced by borderline patients. Using their Dysphoric Affect Scale, a device with which a given patient can be rated on 50 different kinds of mental suffering, they have collected data that provide an objective indication of the pervasiveness, great amplitude, and multifaceted nature of the subjective pain of borderline patients.

Alcoholism

All the principal postmortem studies show many alcoholic persons in cases of completed suicides—about a fourth of all suicides are accounted for by this group (Barraclough et al. 1974; Dorpat and Ripley 1960; Murphy 1992; Robins et al. 1959). Alcoholic persons in particular would appear to be vulnerable to suicide in the managed care environment because of their sensitivity to loss and the danger they will experience excessively brief treatment as an abandonment. In Murphy's (1992) series of alcoholic patients who committed suicide, 41% of the patients had experienced a personal loss

---

[1]Self-hate should be distinguished from low self-esteem. It is possible to hold oneself in low regard without experiencing the malicious, malevolent scorn for oneself that self-hate implies. Self-hate is a much more malignant state.

within 6 weeks of their deaths. I suspect alcoholic patients, especially if depressed, kept in the hospital long enough to "sober up" but discharged to outpatient status with too limited a follow-up plan are at special risk for suicide because they feel abandoned. Indeed, Phillips and colleagues (1998) reported the finding of a 45-fold increase in deaths attributed to the combination of alcohol abuse and medication errors or accidental poisoning in the United States between 1983 and 1993—an increase that coincided with the rise of managed care and shifting of many services to outpatient settings. The alcoholic outpatient is 112.8 times as likely to die from a medication error as are those who are neither outpatients nor alcoholic. To make matters worse, the number of suicides due to alcoholism may well be greater than estimates suggest, because it is likely that many such deaths are classified by the coroners as accidental or due to medication error.

The treatment implication is obvious: Depressed patients, the alcoholic ones especially, should not be discharged to outpatient care with prescriptions that could result in death by accidental or intentional overdosing. These people need extended partial care if a supportive interpersonal net of family or friends is unavailable.

Psychoses

The other principal Axis I disorder found in a significant number of individuals who commit suicide is schizophrenia.[2] The typical schizophrenic suicide completer is a young man about 33 years old who has made a previous attempt and who suffers from a superimposed depression. The patient is likely to have experienced disruption of his personal life because of the corrosive nature of the illness—for example, marital abandonment, threatened or actual loss of other important relationships, loss of employment, rehospitalization, and the like. Severe relapsing episodes seem to predispose to death by suicide (Roy 1986).

The examiner should systematically search for depression in schizophrenic patients and, when it is discovered, treat it vigorously. Warnes (1968) found that three-quarters of his series of schizophrenic patients who committed suicide had depressive symptoms, a finding confirmed by Roy (1982, 1986) and others. Patients with schizoaffective illness are particularly at risk, with the frequency of their suicides rising to the level of patients with major depressive episodes.

---

[2]Barraclough and colleagues (1974) had 3% representation of schizophrenic individuals, Dorpat and Ripley (1960) 11%, and Robins and co-workers (1959) 2% in their postmortem suicide series.

Much has been made of the deadly augury of command hallucinations, namely, auditory hallucinatory voices ordering the patient to kill himself, often in some specific manner (Yager 1989, p. 571). While each patient requires individual study and evaluation, command hallucinations as such are probably an infrequent cause of suicide (Roy 1982, 1986). But psychosis remains a risk factor.

The dark prognosis implied by delusions in a patient with a depressive illness probably has been exaggerated also (Roose et al. 1983). Robins (1986) found that 19% of the 134 subjects who committed suicide were probably psychotic at the time of death—35% of those with affective disorders were delusional, as were 15% of the alcoholic subjects and all three of the schizophrenic subjects.

While most students of suicide agree that delusions heighten the risk for suicide, how significant a risk factor delusions may be is unsettled. Bear in mind that if 35% of the subjects with affective disorder in Robins's study were delusional, the overall prevalence of delusions in patients with bipolar disease is comparable: between 30% and 60% of patients with major affective disorders will be found to have delusions (Goodwin and Jamison 1990, p. 264).

Pitfalls and Snares

The hurried pace of the managed care environment invites certain typical mistakes in the care of suicidal patients. Some of these will now be reviewed from a clinical vantage point; further comment from a risk management view is included in Chapter 8 of this book.

Inadequate History Taking

The hurry to get patients worked up and discharged as briskly as possible makes it easy to overlook the fundamental requirement of good psychiatric care: the taking of a good history. It has been long appreciated that history obtained only from the patient is likely to be incomplete or incorrect. In the current environment, to omit taking a history from family members or others who know the patient well is very tempting. It remains essential to listen closely to what those *other than the patient* have to say and to question them carefully. This is particularly true in cases of treatment-resistant patients who do not want the clinical staff to interfere in their plans for suicide, and when there is psychosis. Failure to get a full history can sometimes lead to misdiagnosis, and misdiagnosis leads to mistreatment.

Case Example

A 23-year-old graduate student was admitted to an inpatient service mute, accompanied by numerous notebooks filled with obviously psychotic material concerning angels and devils. Though there was a strong family history of bipolar disorder, and the patient had had a prior depressive episode, a hurried diagnosis of schizophrenia, catatonic type, was made. No history was taken from the relatives. The diagnosis of depressive stupor [Hoch 1921] was never entertained.

Haloperidol was given and the patient soon seemed better. Noting that the patient's behavior was less bizarre, the staff allowed him to leave the ward on a pass, not grasping that he was dangerously depressed. The patient left the area and hanged himself in a few hours.

If the initial history taking is too rushed or carried out in an unempathic manner, poor rapport will result and the treatment will get off to a bad start.

Case Example

A suspicious and very depressed elderly patient withheld critically important information from her admitting psychiatrist at the time of initial interview. Later, when a consultant asked her why, she snapped, "He was firing questions at me out of that little DSM book right and left just so he could decide what pill to give me, and I couldn't get a word in edgewise."

Failure to Reexamine the Patient Carefully, Especially Before Discharge

Although psychiatrists usually examine new patients carefully at the time of admission, there is a tendency to rely on treatment team reports as discharge approaches, sometimes omitting the vital final interview and mental state examination. Psychiatrists may overlook the fact that much information reported by the staff is based not on systematic interviewing but on casual corridor observation instead. The patient who appears much brighter after a few days' hospital stay may not be all that sunny in the privacy of his own mind. Somebody needs to make sure of his mind before discharge.

It is well to compare what the patient tells the staff about the level of anguish, self-hate, and hopelessness (suicidality) with what he tells friends and family.

Case Example

A 42-year-old woman told her inpatient psychiatrist and the nurses that she was feeling much better and looked forward to leaving the hospital. At the same time, however, she told her outpatient therapist and her husband that she expected to take her life soon and gave them detailed instructions for the dispersal of her cremated body. No exchange of this critical information took place. The patient was discharged and jumped off a high building.

Overlooking Suicidal Shifts in Recovering Patients

The first 6–12 months after discharge is statistically a period of high risk for recovering depressed patients. When inpatient stays average between 5 and 15 days, it is impossible to anticipate and cope with sudden mental state shifts that occur in these individuals except on an outpatient basis. Patients who are recovering from psychotic depressions are particularly unpredictable. These patients are sometimes discharged from the hospital following antipsychotic treatment that clears the psychosis but before depression has lifted.

Furthermore, when a patient is treated with antidepressant medicines or with electroconvulsive therapy for depression, a hypomanic upswing may occur. Should such an upswing evolve into a mixed episode (American Psychiatric Association 1994, p. 335), the suicide danger may increase (Maltsberger 1997). When a paranoid psychosis masking a depression lifts, a suicidal mental state sometimes effloresces (Allen 1967). Unless the outpatient therapist receiving a recovering patient watches out for such developments, he may be taken unawares and lose a patient to suicide.

Case Example

A 50-year-old widow developed a paranoid psychosis with hypomanic features after the death of her husband. Inpatient treatment resulted in the gradual resolution of the excited and aggressive behavior, and an increasingly quiet mental state supervened. The patient was discharged to be followed as an outpatient, but she took a lethal dose of barbiturate a few days later. (Berman et al. 1992)

Obviously, the burden of monitoring the patient closely for any of these suicidal developments falls on the outpatient clinician. These patients must be seen frequently enough after discharge so that changes of this nature may be noticed and treated should they appear. In my opinion, psychotic and bipolar patients should be seen at least weekly for several months after discharge and watched closely. Monthly sessions are too infrequent.

Reliance on "Contracts"

In some hospitals, the staff believe that getting the patient to enter into a "contract" to do no self-harm (sometimes patients are even required to sign such a contract in writing) is an effective suicide preventative. This is simply not so. While a patient should be encouraged to bring rising levels of distress to the attention of staff and to try and let the nurse know if he is feeling more self-injurious, a promise is by no means a guarantee. In fact, such contracting can lull caregivers into a false sense of security. A patient who suddenly feels overwhelmed with agony is likely to forget all about promises of this nature.

Case Example

A woman with borderline personality disorder complicated by treatment-resistant major depression was followed for a number of months as an outpatient. At the end of each session her therapist made her promise that she would not kill herself before their next meeting. She promised as required, but one day when her doctor forgot to extract the usual promise, she went home and made a serious suicide attempt.

Reluctance to Prescribe Electroconvulsive Treatment

Some depressed patients may require 6 weeks to respond to psychopharmacological treatment, and many do not respond until 2 weeks have passed. Inpatient stays now last something like 10 days or less. Electroconvulsive treatment (ECT) is usually followed by distinct clinical improvement after the third session, if not sooner. If initiated early in the hospital stay, this therapy will usually result in substantial improvement by the 10th day.

In the United States, at least, most psychiatrists still prefer to treat suicidally depressed patients with drugs, even though such a course promises slower improvement and, often enough, partial improvement. Patients are sometimes discharged even before the drugs have had a good opportunity to act.

ECT has repeatedly been shown to be effective. With modern anesthetic and treatment techniques, it is very safe. Furthermore, ECT leads to briefer, less expensive inpatient sojourns (Olfson et al. 1998). Indeed, when administered in a timely manner on an outpatient basis, ECT will make many hospital admissions unnecessary.

ECT may well be the treatment of choice for patients with psychotic or deeply suicidal depressions because its rapid effect interrupts the long waiting period drug treatment usually requires—often a long stretch of time during which the patient remains at risk. Obviously, there is much to recommend ECT in the managed care era.

Prejudice against this treatment is deeply entrenched in this country, and the psychiatric profession itself is not free of irrational negative bias. In some parts of the United States, ECT is hardly given at all (Hermann et al. 1995). Some psychiatric residency programs appear to offer little teaching about this life-saving treatment; trainees in such systems perhaps never witness a treatment session (Salzman 1998).

Case Example

A 27-year-old dishwasher fell into a suicidal depression and developed the delusion that his wife had a secret lover. She was worn out and had begun divorce proceedings. The patient was prescribed antipsychotic and antidepressant drugs and appeared to improve over the next several days. He was discharged on the fourth hospital day because his mental state seemed better, though no detailed assessment was recorded in the chart. He killed himself with a shotgun the same afternoon. ECT had not been considered.

Changing From One Clinician to Another

More often than not, the patient who is discharged from inpatient to outpatient status loses the inpatient psychiatrist and must begin afresh with a new doctor. Recently achieved emotional equilibrium based on the support of inpatient staff is tenuous; losing that support on discharge can provoke a worsening of symptoms. Discontinuity of care has been a problem in treating suicidal patients for many years. These patients are particularly prone to feel rejected, and a sense of abandonment can trigger suicide. The greatly increased volume of patients passing through inpatient wards has aggravated the problem. We have empirical evidence that patients with borderline personality disorder and alcohol and drug abuse problems may be *lethally* sensitive to loss and rejection (Kullgren et al. 1986; Murphy 1992).

Discontinuity of care in the transition between inpatient and outpatient status should be avoided whenever possible. When it is not possible, the outpatient clinician should make every effort to meet his patient-to-be several times in order to establish a therapeutic rapport before the protective inpatient relationships are lost.

Case Example

A 35-year-old plumber was admitted to inpatient care because of depression and suicide threats. He was begun on antidepressant medicines. After a few days, he left the hospital before the staff felt he was entirely ready, but the psychiatrist did not feel he met the criteria for involuntary care. The patient was given an appointment to be followed at an outpatient clinic in a week, but the patient did not know who he was to see there. He did not keep the appointment and shortly afterward hanged himself.

Miscommunication

It is obvious that many of the errors outlined here are sprouts that germinate from miscommunication. The era in which the inpatient social worker came to know each patient's family or friends is long past. In the present treatment environment, close communication from and to these important outsiders is often neglected. The nodes where errors in communication are likely to occur are

1. at admission, when history taking is incomplete or faulty;
2. during the course of hospitalization when staff and the patient's significant others need to be talking but are not;
3. when discharge is first planned, a time when full knowledge of the patient's life and circumstances is needed but is lacking;
4. when aftercare needs careful arrangement but does not get it; and
5. when the staff fail to make sure aftercare plans have been followed through.

Though the importance of good record keeping can hardly be exaggerated, even the most meticulous record cannot substitute for oral discussion and information exchange if patients' treatment is to be carried through appropriately.

Conclusion

Good treatment of suicidal patients in the current era of managed care demands careful attention to correct suicide risk assessment. Such assessment rests first and foremost on careful history taking. Attention to correct diagnosis and the treatment of psychic pain that so typically accompanies major mental illness is critically important. Scrupulous attention to matters of communication between staff, between staff and those outsiders close to the patient, between staff and patient, and between staff and those responsible for aftercare will go far in preventing needless suicides.

References

Allen TE: Suicidal impulse in depression and paranoia. Int J Psychoanal 48:433–438, 1967

American Psychiatric Association, Diagnostic and Statistical Manual of Mental Disorders, 4th Edition. Washington, DC, American Psychiatric Association, 1994

American Psychiatric Association, Diagnostic and Statistical Manual of Mental Disorders, 4th Edition, Text Revision. Washington, DC, American Psychiatric Association, 2000

Barraclough B, Bunch J, Nelson B, et al: A hundred cases of suicide: clinical aspects. Br J Psychiatry 125:355–373, 1974

Berman AL, Maltsberger JT, Fenton WS: The suicide of Marigold Perry. Suicide Life Threat Behav 22:396–405, 1992

Dorpat TL, Ripley HS: A study of suicide in the Seattle area. Compr Psychiatry 1:349–359, 1960

Fawcett J: The detection and consequences of anxiety in clinical depression. J Clin Psychiatry 58 (no. 8, suppl):35–40, 1997

Fawcett J, Scheftner WA, Fogg L, et al: Time-related predictors of suicide in major affective disorder. Am J Psychiatry 147:1189–1194, 1990

Goodwin FK, Jamison KR: Manic Depressive Illness. New York, Oxford University Press, 1990

Hermann RC, Dorwart RA, Hoover CW, et al: Variation in ECT use in the United States. Am J Psychiatry 152:869–875, 1995

Hoch A: Benign Stupors. A Study of a New Manic-Depressive Reaction Type. New York, Macmillan, 1921

Kraepelin E: Manic-Depressive Insanity and Paranoia. Translated by Barclay RM; edited by Robertson GM. Edinburgh, E & S Livingston, 1921 [reprinted in facsimile by the Ayer Company, Salem, NH, in 1987]

Kullgren G, Renberg E, Jacobson L: An empirical study of borderline personality disorder and psychiatric suicides. J Nerv Ment Dis 174:328–331, 1986

Lewin R: Managed care and the discharge dilemma. Psychiatry 53:116–121, 1990

Maltsberger JT: Suicide Risk: The Formulation of Clinical Judgment. New York, New York University Press, 1986

Maltsberger JT: Ecstatic suicide. Archives of Suicide Research 3:283–301, 1997

Manasse HR: Increase in US medication-error deaths. Lancet 351:1655 [discussion: 1657), 1998

Maris RW, Berman AL, Maltsberger JT, et al: Assessment and Prediction of Suicide. New York, Guilford, 1992

Mish FC (ed): Webster's Ninth New Collegiate Dictionary. Springfield, MA, Merriam-Webster Co, 1988

Murphy GE. Suicide in Alcoholism. New York, Oxford University Press, 1992

Olfson M, Marcus S, Sackeim HA, et al: The use of ECT for the inpatient treatment of recurrent major depression. Am J Psychiatry 155:22–29, 1998

Phillips DP, Christenfeld N, Glynn LM: Increase in US medication-error deaths between 1983 and 1993. Lancet 351:643–644 [discussion: 1657], 1998

Robins E: Psychosis and suicide. Biol Psychiatry 21:665–672, 1986

Robins E, Murphy GE, Wilkinson SG, et al: Some clinical considerations in the prevention of suicide based on a study of one hundred thirty-four successful suicides. Am J Public Health 49:888–899, 1959

Roose SP, Glassman AH, Walsh T, et al: Depression, delusions, and suicide. Am J Psychiatry 140:1159–1162, 1983

Roy A: Suicide in chronic schizophrenia. Br J Psychiatry 141:171–177, 1982

Roy A: Suicide. Baltimore, MD, Williams & Wilkins, 1986

Salzman C: ECT, research, and professional ambivalence. Am J Psychiatry 155:1–2, 1998

Schouten R: Legal liability and managed care. Harv Rev Psychiatry 1:189–190, 1993

Sharfstein SS: The catastrophic case: a special problem for general hospital psychiatry in the era of managed care. Gen Hosp Psychiatry 11:268–270, 1989

Shneidman ES: Suicide as psychache. J Nerv Ment Dis 181:147–149, 1993

Warnes H: Suicide in schizophrenia. Diseases of the Nervous System 29:35–40, 1968

Westermeyer J: Problems with managed psychiatric care without a psychiatrist-manager. Hospital and Community Psychiatry 2:1221–1224, 1991

Yager J: Clinical manifestations of psychiatric disorders, in Comprehensive Textbook of Psychiatry/V, 5th Edition, Vol 1. Edited by Kaplan HI, Sadock BJ. Baltimore, MD, Williams & Wilkins, 1989, pp 553–582

Zanarini MC, Frankenburg FR, DeLuca CJ, et al: The pain of being borderline: dysphoric affects specific to borderline personality disorder. Harv Rev Psychiatry 6:201–207, 1998

CHAPTER 2

Managed Crisis Care for Suicidal Patients

Judith Feldman, M.D.
Linda Finguerra, R.N., C.S.

F or suicidal patients, their families, and their treaters, "crisis" implies a time not only of danger but also of opportunity. For the patient there is the opportunity to cry for help and to be heard, to break through denial of illness or loss, and to receive support and to learn more about his or her internal conflict or vulnerability. For the family, a crisis provides the opportunity to communicate, to forgive, to forge new alliances, and to reach new levels of understanding. For the clinician, treating a patient through a suicidal crisis may strengthen the therapeutic alliance and allow new material into the therapeutic arena. For all, successful navigation of a suicidal crisis may lay the foundation for future treatment and, ultimately, for the prevention of suicide.

Successful crisis management involves providing access to care, assessing risk appropriately, providing immediate intervention, and laying the groundwork for longer-term care. In this chapter, we outline the major issues involved in providing access, assessing risk, making appropriate treatment decisions, and providing immediate and long-term care to suicidal patients in fee-for-service and managed systems. We discuss the special challenges and opportunities involved in caring for the chronically suicidal patient with a personality disorder. Finally, using the same framework, we describe an approach to crisis management that we have found effective within our managed care setting.

Elements of Suicide Crisis Management

Access

A crisis care system should include rapid access to telephone triage and counseling, ambulance and police services, medical emergency services, and secure psychiatric crisis facilities. Around the country, a variety of suicide "hotlines" and suicide prevention centers have emerged to provide such services. Although there is some controversy about hotlines, suicide prevention centers seem to have had a preventive effect on suicide. One descriptive study (Lester 1993), for example, found an association between the presence of suicide prevention centers in a state and negative changes in the suicide rate from 1970 to 1980. Patients with suicidal ideation or intent may be able to delay self-destructive action if they have prompt access to telephone or face-to-face intervention (Morgan et al. 1993). Family members who discover a patient in the act of a suicide attempt can turn to such services for immediate guidance to help them intervene effectively.

Many patients who commit suicide have already received some psychiatric care. In one study of depressed patients (Fawcett et al. 1993), 50% of individuals who completed suicide were in psychiatric treatment at the time of the suicide, and 50% had seen a physician in the past month. In another study (Roy 1982), 58% had seen a physician during the previous week. Other patients, however, may enter the mental health system for the first time during a suicidal crisis and may not know how to get access to emergency care. Strong suicidal urges may persist for relatively short periods of time, even in patients with chronic suicidal ideation, so easily accessed, prompt intervention may be needed to prevent acute self-harm.

Easy access to follow-up care may also have a preventive effect. A British controlled trial (Morgan et al. 1993) demonstrated that patients who were offered rapid access to on-call trainee psychiatrists after an episode of deliberate self-harm made fewer subsequent attempts and placed less demand on medical services than did control subjects.

Assessment

We view the primary task of suicide crisis assessment as the need to determine the appropriate level of care for immediate treatment. To accomplish this task, crisis evaluation of a suicidal patient should yield a reliable estimate of the likelihood of serious self harm. Many states use the phrase "likelihood of serious harm" in statutes that justify civil commitment for psychiatric illness. A clinician evaluating a particular patient needs to evaluate an individual's risk *at that moment,* taking into account the patient's current and past history, data provided by additional informants, psychiatric diagnostic assessment, and relevant demographic factors that may heighten risk.

Various methods and guidelines have been developed for this assessment, including the dimensions of intent and lethality (Jacobs 1982), measurement of hopelessness in depressed patients (Beck et al. 1990), a multiaxial assessment framework (Risk Management Foundation 1996), and the "formulation of suicide risk" (see Appendix B, this volume). Establishing a DSM diagnosis is helpful in this process because of the known association of specific diagnoses with increased risk (see Chapter 1, this volume), but patients of all diagnoses may commit suicide. Therefore, in this chapter on crisis intervention, we focus more directly on the process of understanding the "suicide crisis" while keeping the psychiatric diagnosis in mind as an additional factor that influences treatment decisions.

Structured rating scales may allow the evaluator and patient to quantify suicide risk. Multiaxial rating systems such as the Patient Assessment Tool (Harvard Pilgrim Health Care 1996) hold some promise but have not been extensively tested for predictive value. In a prospective study of 1,958 depressed outpatients (Beck et al. 1990), the Beck Hopelessness Scale score was significantly related to eventual suicide.

Although as yet no published scale or guideline has been shown to predict future dangerousness accurately or to dictate a precise level of care, some evidence suggests that trained emergency room clinicians do in fact arrive at consistent decisions when evaluating dangerousness and the need for civil commitment. In one study of 251 cases in public emergency rooms in California (Segal et al. 1988), the investigators found that an independent assessment that used an index of behavioral indicators (danger to self or others, grave disability) and a concurrent measure of perceived dangerousness predicted admission decisions of 70 clinicians.

Various authors (Jacobs 1982; Linehan 1993a) have stressed the need for the clinician to examine his or her own responses to the patient, suggesting that annoyance, hate, hopelessness, fear, pity, or indifference may make it difficult for the clinician to assess dangerousness. These emotions may also be used, by the trained psychotherapist, as a mirror of the experience of the patient and may be helpful in understanding the patient and in forming an alliance. Whereas the subjective feeling of "risk" may alert a clinician that a patient is in danger, a subjective feeling of "safety" or "good alliance" is not necessarily to be trusted in an assessment of dangerousness.

Consideration of validated demographic risk factors can sharpen the accuracy of suicide crisis evaluations (see Appendix A, this volume). One prospective 10-year study of suicide risk in depressed patients (Fawcett et al. 1993) revealed two distinct groups of predictive variables. Those who committed suicide during the year following evaluation were characterized by panic attacks, impaired concentration, agitation, moderate alcohol use, and severe anhedonia. Those who completed suicide 2–10 years after evaluation were characterized at entry by severe hopelessness and a history of suicide attempts. What distinguished the patients who committed suicide as a group from the those who did not were the former's freedom from responsibility for children and the presence of cycling affective illness, particularly when comorbid with drug or alcohol abuse.

Although Fawcett et al.'s findings were derived from a study of depressed patients, we consider it prudent for the clinician to pay special attention to symptoms of panic, agitation, alcohol use, and cycling affective illness in any potentially suicidal patient. In addition, there is considerable agreement that the presence of a serious psychiatric illness (Fawcett et al. 1993; Jacobs 1982; Roy 1982), a history of previous suicide attempts (Fawcett et al. 1993; Jacobs 1982), substance use disorders (Beautrais et al. 1996; Fawcett et al. 1993; Jacobs 1982), or comorbidity (Beautrais et al. 1996) are positive correlates of suicide risk. Patients with personality disorders who complete suicide are almost always found to have current depressive syndromes, substance use disorders, or both (Isometsa et al. 1996). Although the classic demographic profile of a suicide completer as a male, over age 45, living alone, not married, and unemployed remains valid (Fawcett et al. 1993; see also Appendix A, this volume), these statistical correlates should not deceive the clinician into overlooking the significant risk of suicide among adolescents and young adults (see Chapter 6, this volume).

Assessment of the chronically or repeatedly suicidal patient poses a special challenge. These patients often meet the criteria for severe personality disorders as well as substance use disorders (Ennis et al. 1985). They may present repeatedly to emergency rooms and may be difficult to engage in treatment, evoking feelings of dislike and frustration among clinicians (Bassuk and Gerson 1980; Ellison et al.1986). They often also engage in repeated self-harming (termed *parasuicidal*) behavior (Kreitman 1976), such as cutting, scratching, or burning themselves, making it difficult to assess immediate risk against the background of chronic despair and self-injurious behavior. Though the clinician may feel safer or more prudent hospitalizing such a patient, a hospitalization may purchase immediate safety at the expense of reinforcing maladaptive coping strategies. This can promote regression that will prove detrimental to long-term progress (Linehan 1993a).

The emergency use of a "no-harm contract" is more appropriately discussed as a tool of assessment (see Chapter 1, this volume) than of intervention, because its most valuable use is in exploring a patient's capacity to participate in a therapeutic alliance. Stanford and colleagues (1994) reviewed the literature on these contracts from a diagnostic, therapeutic, and medicolegal perspective. They concluded that the no-harm contract provides no reliable assurance that a patient will be safe from suicide. Its use, indeed, can inadvertently give false reassurance to patient and clinician, interfering with a more appropriate assessment and disposition process. It is never legally binding, and sometimes it is entered into with patients who lack competency to understand such an agreement in any case.

Immediate Intervention

The beginning of intervention is the assessment itself. An explication of the factors leading up to the crisis, an inventory of environmental supports and the patient's ability to use these supports, and a discussion of impasses in treatment can help the patient gain understanding and feel less overwhelmed and helpless. Once the patient understands why she or he became more suicidal, intervention should focus on concrete plans to cope with the crisis. Clinician and patient together should discuss coping strategies; engage family, friends, and therapist as appropriate; and make contingency plans if suicidal impulses should reemerge. The patient's ability to work with the clinician on this plan may influence the decision about which level of care is most appropriate.

In the context of a suicide crisis, immediate intervention includes medical assessment and treatment, psychiatric assessment and treatment, and disposition. The assessment and intervention processes may involve several different levels of care depending on the clinical situation. Some suicidal crises, for example with a patient in a well-established psychotherapy, can be handled safely with a telephone conversation. Some require a face-to-face evaluation. Others (particularly in adolescent patients) may require a family evaluation or the gathering of information from informants in addition to the patient. The prescription of pharmacotherapeutic agents may be a part of this immediate intervention (but is not the focus of this chapter; see Chapter 7 for a fuller discussion) in the presence of psychosis, intolerable anxiety, agitation, noncompliance with a preexisting medication regimen, toxicity from prescribed medications, or withdrawal symptoms following use of recreational drugs.

The locus of assessment can be tailored to the patient's individual needs, following a general principle that higher-risk circumstances warrant more intensive assessment settings. Any patient with a suspected overdose or altered state of consciousness should be transported immediately (usually by ambulance, since moving a confused or psychotic patient can be very hazardous) to an emergency room for diagnosis and medical treatment. Patients who have already attempted suicide should be assumed to need medical care in an emergency room or intensive care unit in addition to a psychiatric assessment.

For patients who do not require intensive medical stabilization or monitoring, treatment modalities in immediate intervention may include observation, detoxification, medication, or intensive individual and/or family counseling. This care may be given in an emergency room, a crisis center, or an overnight holding area, or as a home-based intervention. Disposition may involve admission to a locked hospital unit, a partial hospital program, an outpatient setting, a shelter, or a residential treatment center. Unfortunately, no clear guidelines are yet available to match specific patients, presenting problems, risk factors, and psychosocial support systems to unique levels and modalities of care.

Crisis clinicians are sometimes surprised to learn how few studies have assessed the outcome effects of suicide crisis intervention. A recent pooled analysis of controlled studies of suicide attempters showed no significant effect of psychosocial crisis intervention, guaranteed shelter, or treatment of poor compliance on repeat suicide attempts. Cognitive-behavioral approaches, however, were shown in four studies to significantly reduce the likelihood of future attempts (van der Sande et al. 1997). Further research in this area is sorely needed.

Laying the Groundwork for Longer-Term Care

Successful navigation of a crisis is often the beginning of more definitive treatment. For some patients, a suicidal crisis is the first contact with psychiatric care. The suicidal patient may form a meaningful bond with the first mental health professional who sees her. This clinician must be careful to inform the patient, therefore, whether he can continue with her treatment or will refer her to another therapist. When referral is necessary, it should be done with care. It is valuable to contact the referred patient subsequently to ensure that a follow-up appointment is kept and that the treatment plan is experienced as satisfactory.

Whenever a suicidal patient is already associated with one or more mental health providers, the crisis clinician should communicate with these ongoing treaters about his findings, including precipitants to the current crisis, mental status, risk assessment, and recommendations for immediate and ongoing care. The crisis assessment can be a valuable consultation to the ongoing treatment team, and clinicians already familiar with the patient can often shed light on the nature of an acute regression. A patient's reluctance to give consent for such communication may signify a problem in the treatment or indicate the patient's more general distrust of her caregivers.

A patient in ongoing treatment (often both psychotherapy and pharmacotherapy) will often return to her previous treatment relationship(s) after contact with a crisis clinician to further address the issues which led to the crisis. The crisis may have been precipitated by a perceived problem in the treatment relationship, ineffectiveness of a pharmacotherapeutic regimen, or difficulties with side effects in the pharmacotherapy, leading to noncompliance and reemergence of psychiatric symptoms. A suicide attempt may signify the patient's experience of a breach of trust between psychotherapist and patient, such as the patient's failure to reach out or the psychotherapist's failure to respond in a way that helped the patient feel attended to. Such a breach requires working through in order to accomplish repair of the alliance.

The response of a clinician and treatment system to a patient in crisis will set the tone for the patient's expectations regarding the handling of future crises. A patient who is always sent to a hospital will anticipate hospitalization. A patient who always receives extra sessions with her therapist will anticipate extra sessions. Such contingencies may or may not be consistent with the goals of other concurrent components of treatment and therefore should be considered carefully in each individual case.

While admission to a locked psychiatric unit with constant observation is never completely effective in preventing a suicide, the safety and containment of a psychiatric hospital may be life-saving for some patients; however, many patients will benefit from participating in less-restrictive treatment plans. Not every patient who expresses suicidal ideation should be hospitalized. Patients with severe personality disorders often regress in an inpatient setting when their abrogation of responsibility for their own safety is inadvertently rewarded and reinforced by intense clinical support and attention (Maltsberger 1994). For patients with repeated crises, hospitalization may in fact increase the likelihood of future behaviors that undermine more definitive recovery.

Case Example

A 37-year-old homosexual man with recurrent major depressive disorder and a history of sexual trauma made a highly lethal suicide attempt after precipitously leaving his partial hospital program. When he returned to the partial hospital after an inpatient stay and later became suicidal, he was hospitalized against his will by the partial hospital staff. The following year, when he had another suicidal episode, he was reluctant to call the crisis unit for fear he would be committed to the hospital—an experience he had found distasteful and shameful. He did call, however. The clinician he met with reviewed the onset of his suicidal ideation and helped him to trace it back to a fight with his lover and his anger at his lover's unwillingness to make a commitment to him. The patient experienced relief at this realization and stated that he no longer felt suicidal. After careful reassessment of the patient, the crisis clinician felt that he could return home and be seen the following day. When the patient reflected later on this crisis encounter, he said, "I liked Laura's approach; she doesn't commit people, she talks to them." The crisis clinician clarified that sometimes she does commit people, but talks to them first, and hopes that if a hospitalization is indicated, it can be a voluntary one.

Managed Care

Treatment of the suicidal patient in a managed care system[1] may present unique advantages but also poses unique problems. In a good managed care system, care is well organized and coordinated, all levels of care are accessible, case management is used to ensure continuity of care, clinical information is available as appropriate, and medical and mental health care

---

[1]*Managed systems* are organized care systems that accept premium dollars and bear financial risk for care. They either provide the care themselves or contract with delivery systems who provide the care. The following terms are frequently encountered in discussions of managed systems: IPA (independent practice association): a network of primary care physicians, working in private offices, capitated for care of a population of patients. Mental health services in an IPA are usually "carved out" to a mental health management company. PPO (preferred provider organization): an insurance product in which members are covered for care in a network of "preferred providers" but may see a provider outside the network by paying more (higher copay, deductibles, or more limited coverage). HMO (health maintenance organization): a managed care company that accepts a capitation for its members and provides care through a closed group of salaried clinicians working in buildings in organized departments. POS (point-of-service): a PPO product in which members can decide at each point-of-service whether to go to a preferred or nonpreferred provider. MEP (managed entitlement plan): a managed system that accepts dollars from a federal or state entitlement plan (Medicare, Medicaid) and manages the care using an IPA, PPO, or HMO.

complement each other. In their efforts to conserve resources, however, managed systems run the risk of undertreatment; furthermore, many of these systems are large ones, in which some patients may "fall between the cracks" or encounter bureaucratic roadblocks to care. In the following section, we detail the benefits and alert the clinician to problems of a managed system in providing suicide crisis care.

Access

If patients belong to a managed care plan (IPA, preferred provider organization [PPO], HMO, point-of-service [POS] plan, or managed entitlement plan [MEP]), they theoretically have automatic access to coverage for care. Most managed care plans designate specific systems of access. These include toll-free numbers, primary care "gatekeeping," or a closed panel of providers or crisis centers. Although these systems may help a patient determine whom to call in a crisis, they may also be experienced as barriers to care if, for example, the patient is put "on hold" too long by the access line or is unable to reach his or her or primary care physician. A staff model HMO, with salaried providers and a "clinic" setting, will often have an emergency clinician available during working hours and some combination of an on-call clinician and a crisis center after hours. This kind of a system can facilitate access to a skilled clinician but may also make it more difficult for a patient in active treatment to access his or her own psychotherapist during a crisis.

An important advantage of a managed system is the availability of primary care and emergency medical services for plan members and their families. Systems of access to medical care (including ambulance transportation) and communication between medical and mental health clinicians can increase the quality and efficiency of crisis care for suicidal patients. On the other hand, a patient who belongs to an IPA or PPO may be in treatment with a contracted clinician who sees the patient in a private office but must contact the managed care company if the patient requires crisis care or hospitalization. The clinician, attempting to secure more intensive treatment for a patient, may find himself or herself in an interaction with a utilization manager who does not know the patient and may be advocating for a less intense, less costly level of care. This situation, if well managed, could end up providing helpful consultation to a clinician frustrated by the repetitive crises of a patient with a personality disorder. If the utilization manager is skilled, creative, and free to act on the basis of medical necessity, he or she may be able to offer solutions not available to the office-based therapist (e.g., respite beds and home care) in order to keep the patient out of the hospital. However, the managed care precertification process may serve as a bureaucratic barrier, delaying care in an urgent situation. The situation is even more complicated if the treating clinician is not affiliated with the managed care company. Lazarus (1993) presents a case series in which emergency care is delayed or complicated by disagreements between outpatient clinician, emergency clinician, and managed care representative. For helpful strategies in dealing with utilization managers, see the discussion of clinical guidelines later in this chapter and in Appendix B at the end of this book.

In providing access to care, an unmanaged system has the advantages that a patient's access to care is less restricted, more frequent emergency contact with his or her own psychotherapist may be covered, and there may be fewer barriers to hospitalization. A managed system has the advantages of available case consultation, alternatives to hospitalization, case management, coverage for crisis care, and better coordination with primary care medicine. For suggestions on how to gain access to these resources, see the discussion of clinical guidelines later in this chapter.

Assessment

A managed system of care that possesses an efficient system of records and communication offers the possibility that information may be shared efficiently between clinicians. This communication is enhanced by its limiting the choice of designated hospitals and crisis centers available to its members. Outpatient clinicians can phone or fax the appropriate crisis center to file and update current information about a patient's risk, current stressors, ongoing treatment plan, or behavioral contracts (see the discussion of clinical guidelines later in this chapter). The clinician can be fairly confident that his or her patient will receive crisis care at that crisis center, since it is the only one authorized by the managed care system. In many managed systems, crisis centers also have direct access to automated medical records. While each suicide crisis situation must be assessed anew, the availability of clinical information is usually quite helpful in making an accurate assessment. In addition, expert or collegial consultations are often made readily available to clinicians within an organized system. Many managed systems also have on-call lawyers or forensic psychiatrists who may be helpful in a suicide crisis evaluation (see the discussion of clinical guidelines later in this chapter).

Large systems of care may dilute clinical responsibility. A solo practitioner who is managing a suicidal patient bears all the risk and all the anxiety. Under these circumstances, it is possible that a solo practitioner would be more likely to reach out to a patient. However, there are no studies yet

Managed Crisis Care for Suicidal Patients

demonstrating that suicidal patients in managed care systems receive less aggressive outreach that those in fee-for-service care. This is an area worthy of research.

Immediate Intervention

One of the fundamental tenets of managed mental health care is provision of care in the least intensive, least restrictive setting appropriate to the clinical situation. In order to conserve resources and provide optimal care of a population, a managed system of care will attempt to find this "least restrictive" level for each patient as he or she presents for treatment. This has advantages and disadvantages for the crisis care of the suicidal patient.

One advantage is that the managed system is quite likely to develop, or to contract with, a fairly complete spectrum of services for its members. In addition to inpatient and outpatient care, managed care systems may include partial hospital programs, acute residential treatment centers, crisis centers, holding beds, respite care, shelters, emergency foster care, and home assessment and intervention services. Effective managed systems will have developed criteria for admission to each level of care and a utilization management process for admitting patients and providing continuity as they move from one level of care to another (see the discussion of clinical guidelines later in this chapter). The larger and better organized the system, the more likely that specialists will be available to manage crises and provide the appropriate modality of treatment. It is a great advantage to have child and family therapists, behavior therapists, addictions specialists, and skilled crisis clinicians available to intervene with patients in suicidal crises and to consult with the clinicians who care for them on an ongoing basis.

Disadvantages of a managed system include the risk that a patient will be undertreated, discharged too early, or placed in less restrictive levels of care than are needed for adequate safety. The managed system as a whole, however, must provide care, with fixed resources, to an entire population. Therefore, the incentives are toward shorter treatment and less use of hospitals when clinically appropriate.[2] Whether suicide risk from undertreatment

---

[2]This is a very complicated issue. A *fee-for-service system of care* is one in which clinicians and hospitals receive more money the more care they give and a clinician's priority is the health and safety of the individual patient. A *managed system* is one in which care must be given to a population within fixed resources and the clinician must balance the responsibility toward the individual patient with the conservation of resources for the covered population as a whole (Sabin 1994). In a *for-profit managed system,* the organization may improve profits, at least in the short term, by providing less costly care.

is greater in managed care systems is an issue that demands further research. An unpublished study suggests that the suicide rate in our specific managed system (Harvard Community Health Plan) is no greater than that in the community it serves (S. Stelovich, J. Harburger, personal communication, 1995), while Lurie and colleagues (1992) reported a suicide rate in a capitated system that was 7% higher than the rate in a fee-for-service system.

For the chronically suicidal patient who may regress in the hospital, a managed system may conceivably provide better care and more recovery over the long term, since the incentives toward cost-containment will increase the likelihood of placement in a less regressive outpatient setting. A 1997 study of clinician assessment of suicide risk of 241 patients on admission and discharge demonstrated that clinicians felt that hospitalization affected variables related to short-term suicide risk but had little effect on variables related to long-term risk (McNiel and Binder 1997). However, there are no studies contrasting the short- and long-term outcomes of crisis treatment of suicidal patients in managed versus unmanaged systems of care.

Managed systems also offer the potential for using guidelines or algorithms for utilization management and clinical decision-making (see, e.g., Risk Management Foundation 1996). Such guidelines or algorithms could reduce variability and ultimately improve the quality of care. Kirstein and co-authors (1975) presented a method to develop operational criteria for utilization review of hospitalization of suicide attempters. Using multiple regression analysis, the authors delineated four predictors for hospitalization: suicide risk, thought disorder, serious intent, and major medical effects of the attempt. Out of 274 charts reviewed retrospectively, only 51 were judged to have shown undertreatment or overtreatment according to these criteria.

It is hoped that evidence-based clinical guidelines can be developed to help managed systems make clinical decisions that would reduce cost without affecting quality. Rissmiller and colleagues (1994) reviewed the literature on factors impeding cost-containment in the treatment of suicidal patients and identified five: lack of a specific, cost-effective screening method to determine true risk of suicide; high number of parasuicidal patients; revolving-door admissions of involuntary patients who become noncompliant with treatment after discharge; discriminatory mental health benefits; and providers' fears of liability. The authors pointed out the low frequency of completed suicides relative to attempts and ideation and emphasized that most inpatients labeled "suicidal" are hospitalized unnecessarily. They recommended managing the care by reserving inpatient treatment for those of high lethality (i.e., high risk at the time of assessment) or those with suicidal ideation plus other risk factors. Other patients could be treated within a service network that would include partial hospitalization and outpatient alternatives. The clinician is still left with the difficult task of determining whether the patient truly demonstrates "high lethality" at the time of assessment.

Laying the Groundwork for Longer-Term Care

In a managed system, it is crucial to understand the meaning of a suicidal crisis and the response of the treatment system to the crisis. Since patients' anticipation of treatment derives from past experience, it is important to establish clear and consistent treatment plans. A plan needs to be responsive to the short- and long-term needs of the individual patient while also taking into account the constraints of the managed system. Provision of high-quality managed crisis care would necessitate a system that could 1) discriminate the patient at current high suicide risk from the chronically suicidal or parasuicidal patient with a personality disorder and 2) balance the wish for immediate safety with the long-term goal of modifying behavior toward appropriate, nonregressive self-management.

Case Example

A 35-year-old patient with posttraumatic stress disorder and parasuicidal behaviors was frequently hospitalized as a consequence of her self-inflicted cuts. During each admission she would regain control for several days but then become more weepy and regressed, unable to get out of bed, clinging to staff and terrified to leave the hospital. After she became a member of a managed entitlement plan, her presentation at the crisis service led to a discussion with her managed care company. The insurer refused to authorize another admission. Her psychotherapist contacted the insurer's case manager, saying he agreed with this decision in the long run but felt that it might be dangerous to the patient to deny hospitalization altogether in the middle of a suicidal crisis. After a discussion that included the psychotherapist and crisis clinician, the patient was approved for a brief admission. She accepted this and understood that a future goal was to reduce the reliance on hospitalization as a means of intervening in her self-destructive behavior episodes.

Effective Managed Crisis Care

In this section, we outline the considerations for providing effective crisis care within a managed system. These issues apply whether the clinician treating a suicidal patient is an independent vendor contracting for the managed care of a population or a private practitioner with no managed care affiliations except through clients who are insured through an HMO, IPA, or PPO. In either case, when the clinician is working with a patient who has a history of suicide attempts, suicidal ideation, or parasuicide, he or she should investigate at the beginning of treatment what services will be available to the patient should a suicide crisis emerge.

In order to provide effective managed crisis care to the suicidal patient, the clinician needs to capitalize on the advantages of the managed system (coordination, available alternatives, consultation and case management, use of guidelines) and minimize the disadvantages (bureaucratic barriers to care, potential undertreatment, dilution of clinical responsibility). In addition, an effective managed crisis system could incorporate clinical guidelines and approaches that might be helpful in distinguishing the chronically suicidal or parasuicidal patient from the patient in an acute, high-risk situation.

Access

In an effective managed system, patients presenting with a suicidal crisis have immediate access to a skilled assessment and an intervention at the appropriate level of care to ensure the most favorable and least costly short- and long-term outcomes. Managed systems usually include emergency psychiatric services that offer a full spectrum of treatment options (e.g., phone triage, face-to-face evaluations, and holding bed capacity) and have the capability of averting unnecessary and prolonged inpatient stays.

Managed care systems concerned about quality improvement issues need to be aware of delays in providing immediate access to emergency psychiatric services, particularly when there is some question about an individual's safety. As Lazarus (1993) pointed out, "[C]linicians and administrators should err on the side of the patient rather than cost containment" (p. 1136). An effective managed system sets standards for access to emergency care and periodically measures and monitors trends in access. It also creates a culture that emphasizes service to individual patients, rewarding clerical as well as clinical staff for quick and empathic responses to patients in crisis.

Assessment

A well-integrated managed crisis system provides algorithms or protocols to guide clinicians' assessment of suicide risk. Validated rating scales, such as the Beck Hopelessness Scale (Beck et al. 1990), or a more "home grown" instrument may be used to support the clinician's assessment. An important strength of managed systems is the capacity for coordination of standards of care among clinicians, within one site and across different sites, so that a shared set of criteria for risk assessment can be agreed upon and applied consistently. A crisis unit associated with Kaiser Permanente used an unvalidated 10-point lethality scale to assess patients who were entering the crisis unit and found that the scale was able to predict which patients were sent home and which were held overnight. When the scale was reapplied the next morning, the score could distinguish those who were admitted from those who were discharged to outpatient care (G. Manning, personal communication, 1993).

Acutely suicidal patients and chronically suicidal patients pose different challenges. In the acute situation, the clinician must perform a careful suicide assessment. If the clinician determines that hospitalization is necessary, he or she must present a case to the case manager or reviewer to authorize admission (see the discussion of clinical guidelines later in this chapter for advice on negotiating this process). An adversarial situation may evolve in which the clinician wants to provide more care and the reviewer wants to provide less care. A more complicated situation is posed by the chronically suicidal patient with a personality disorder. In this case, the same careful assessment is called for, but a decision to hospitalize must be made in the context of the effect of repeated hospitalization on long-term progress and outcome.

Jacobs (1982), in writing about the evaluation and treatment of the suicidal patient within an emergency setting, observed that "because the etiology of a suicidal state is so varied, persons must be diagnosed on the basis of how hard they have been hit, where they can obtain their support, and why they want to live" (p. 364). Even when the patient is a familiar "repeat visitor," with multiple hospitalizations and a known chronic course, careful assessment of the current suicide risk must occur before an inpatient hospitalization can be ruled out (Ellison et al. 1986).

Immediate Intervention

In an effective managed system, medical and mental health care are well integrated. The patient with urgent needs should be able to meet with an appropriately specialized mental health clinician, at the proper level of care, rapidly and conveniently as soon as medical dangers are assessed and/or addressed. For the patient whose suicide attempt was seriously life threatening, medical or psychiatric hospitalization is an almost inevitable disposition. For patients at lesser immediate risk, a well-managed system provides other levels of care (partial hospital, respite care, home-based services, intensive outpatient treatment) and a consistent set of protocols to guide the clinician in determining the appropriate disposition. The information-gathering and transferring possibilities of a coordinated system allow for crisis centers to be in possession of treatment information, including past dispositions and outcomes, and to involve relevant care providers in the development of a new disposition plan.

Laying the Groundwork for Longer-Term Care

For the acutely suicidal patient who returns after a crisis to his or her previous level of functioning, the managed system may offer no real advantage. In fact, it may prove disadvantageous in encouraging time-limited or intermittent care for those patients who may need an ongoing treatment relationship. The promise of an effective managed system is in improvement of ongoing care of the chronically and repeatedly suicidal individual.

Over the past several years, we have explored treatment approaches that offer both patient and clinician an opportunity to understand more clearly the dynamics that catapult a patient toward repetitive crises and suicidal behavior. We have found that incorporating cognitive-behavioral treatment strategies into our treatment spectrum has helped with the management of the chronically suicidal patient. Reinecke (1994) described a cognitive-behavioral approach to crisis management of the suicidal patient. He emphasized that this orientation to treatment

> is multidimensional and acknowledges the importance of behavioral, affective, social and environmental factors in suicide. Cognitive interventions include rational responding, thought monitoring, cognitive distraction, guided imagery, thought stopping, self instruction scaling, guided association, reattribution and examination of idiosyncratic meanings. Behavioral interventions are directed primarily toward developing coping skills, and they include assertiveness or relaxation training, graded task assignments, mastery and pleasure ratings, behavioral rehearsal, in vivo exposure and bibliotherapy. (p. 85)

Recent reviews of the literature on psychotherapy of suicidal individuals (Linehan 1997; van der Sande et al. 1997) suggest that cognitive-behavioral approaches may decrease the frequency of suicide attempts and parasuicidal episodes in some chronically or repeatedly suicidal patients. Especially promising is dialectical behavior therapy (DBT), the systematized variant of cognitive-behavioral treatment developed by Marsha Linehan for the treatment of chronically suicidal patients with borderline personality disorder (see the section on clinical guidelines later in this chapter for a discussion of coverage and authorization for DBT). Linehan conducted two randomized clinical trials of DBT vs "treatment as usual" (Linehan et al. 1991, 1993) which demonstrated that borderline subjects participating in DBT showed a significant decrease in parasuicidal behavior and had fewer inpatient days during the studied interval.

DBT is described by Linehan (1987) as a

> biosocial theory that views parasuicide as problem solving behavior emitted to cope with or ameliorate psychic distress brought on by negative emotional events, self-generated dysfunctional behaviors, and individual temperamental characteristics. Parasuicidal behavior occurs when the individual believes that an intolerable, inescapable life problem exists and that parasuicide is the only or best possible solution; that is the parasuicidal act is regarded as a potentially effective problem solving behavior. (p. 329)

The term *dialectic,* as it is used in DBT, refers to the balance and synthesis of internal opposite poles related to thinking, emotions, and behavior. Both patient and therapist use DBT techniques as a way of *accepting* where the patient is in the moment while moving toward *change*. Treatment strategies integrates cognitive behavior therapy elements with the Eastern concept of *mindfulness*. This eclectic combination of tools helps patients acquire skills that reduce self-injurious behaviors that interfere with treatment and diminish the quality of life. DBT is an organized approach, using standard elements and protocols. As such, it lends itself to an organized system of care such as a clinic, hospital, or managed care setting.

DBT provides a framework for understanding repeated self-injurious behavior as the patient's learned, maladaptive way of coping with emotional pain that the patient may perceive as unbearable. Recasting the patient's vexing behavior in this formulation reduces clinicians' frustration and points the way toward helpful interventions.

After obtaining relevant history, assessing the need for medical intervention, and considering demographic risk factors that may alter treatment approaches, a clinician trained in DBT can intervene with a chronically suicidal patient by using the following DBT elements: behavioral analysis, reinforcement and teaching of new coping skills, and contingency management.

Behavioral Analysis

Behavioral analysis in DBT is a step-by-step assessment of a problematic targeted behavior, focusing on all aspects and circumstances of the behavior, including the antecedents and consequences. In DBT certain behaviors, particularly in the first stage of treatment, are identified as problematic and marked as areas where change is indicated. The hierarchy of goals during the first stage of DBT treatment is 1) decreasing suicidal and/or parasuicidal behavior, 2) decreasing therapy-interfering behaviors, 3) decreasing behaviors that interfere with quality of life, and 4) increasing skills. The patient and clinician closely examine the problematic behavior, precipitants, consequences, and solutions. In this collaboration, the patient is being asked to solve his or her own problem rather than have the environment take over.

In a detailed DBT behavioral analysis, the patient is asked to

1. Describe in specific terms the PROBLEM behavior (what was said, done, thought, or felt).
2. Describe the specific PRECIPITATING event that started the whole chain of behavior.
3. Describe VULNERABILITY factors.
4. Describe in excruciating detail the CHAIN OF EVENTS that led up to the problem behavior.
5. Describe the CONSEQUENCES of this behavior.
6. Describe different SOLUTIONS to the problem.
7. Describe in detail PREVENTION strategy for how patient could have kept the chain from starting by reducing his or her vulnerability to the chain.
8. Describe the REPAIRS that will be done to important or significant consequences of the problem behavior.

The use of behavioral analysis, though time consuming, helps clinician and patient to grasp more fully what factors led up to the suicidal behavior. It also helps them to determine where to go from there, laying the groundwork for appropriate disposition planning and follow-up treatment.

Application of Skills

Linehan (1993b) has described four areas of skills necessary to manage and prevent self-injurious behaviors: mindfulness, interpersonal effectiveness, emotion regulation, and distress tolerance. These skills are outlined in more detail in Linehan's publications, particularly the workbook that accompanies her text (Linehan 1993b).

Clinicians working with chronically suicidal individuals should learn the distress tolerance skills, in particular the crisis survival strategies. These are techniques for helping the patient "hang on" in the face of intolerable affect. They involve distraction, self-soothing, and acceptance.

Linehan emphasizes in her writings that learning new skills in an emotional state is very challenging and that generalizing those skills outside the learning situation is even more difficult. Emergency psychiatric services can use printed handouts from the Linehan skills workbook (Linehan 1993b) to help patients learn these concepts and practice them. The crisis clinician and patient can construct a personalized list of coping strategies for the patient to take with her when she leaves.

Case Example

A patient diagnosed with posttraumatic stress disorder and borderline personality disorder who had been referred to the crisis service for suicidal ideation and self-injurious behavior agreed to do a behavioral analysis. Initially, she reported she had no idea why she cuts herself or feels suicidal. The crisis clinician explained to the patient that it is often helpful to describe in detail the steps leading up to the self-destructive act. The patient, after some attempts to change the subject, began to talk about the chain of events that occurred before she noticed feeling suicidal. The precipitant reported was feeling cut off by her therapist during a session. She then felt increasingly overwhelmed, leading eventually to parasuicidal behavior. The crisis clinician, aware that the parasuicidal behavior was the patient's attempt at managing her emotions, coached the patient around use of emotion regulation, distress tolerance, and interpersonal effectiveness skills. The patient, with support and validation, was able to begin exploring how to commit to the practice of these skills when feeling overwhelmed.

Contingency Management

An effective crisis system should reinforce adaptive behaviors and extinguish problem behaviors. In most systems, the opposite occurs. Patients who self-harm have instant access to high-intensity services; their calls are never put on "hold" when suicide is threatened. These responses can inadvertently reinforce the suicidal behavior. Linehan (1993a) notes that chronically suicidal patients are often under the influences of both operant and respondent behavior. A challenge for any clinician is to respond in a way that both "reduces the eliciting behaviors and minimally reinforces the behavior" (Linehan 1993a).

In a formal DBT treatment contract, patients agree to work on self-harm behavior. They are encouraged to call their therapist at any time, but *before* they harm themselves. After self-harm, they cannot contact their therapists for a brief time period (24–48 hours), though in most instances the patient is aware of backup support. Furthermore, their treatment contract states that a certain number of absences from group or individual treatment may mean termination. This means that being in the hospital puts their valuable treatment in jeopardy.

For appropriately selected patients, a crisis unit should replicate these contingencies whenever possible. Patients should get encouragement and reinforcement for calling before self-harming. A call after a parasuicidal act should elicit a brief dangerousness assessment and a behavioral analysis.

Case Example

A borderline patient told the crisis clinician that she cut herself the evening she was discharged from the day hospital: "They didn't understand how depressed I was," she said. "They just wanted me to get on with things. I was so overwhelmed that I cut myself and I don't see any point in living if I can't get support." The usual scenario would involve a struggle between the managed care crisis clinician's attempts to "set limits" and "avoid regression" by sending the patient home, and the patient's ever more desperate attempts to show the clinician how miserable she is.

The dialectic approach, by contrast, would balance the crisis clinician's validation of the patient's misery, fear, and feelings of abandonment with the clarification that the patient had agreed to work on diminishing her self-harm behavior and handle these feelings using her DBT skills. A behavioral analysis would help clarify where the patient lost that focus, and what she could have done to modify her emotions, tolerate her distress, or negotiate more effectively for an acceptable discharge plan.

Clinical Guidelines

The following guidelines may be helpful to the clinician who is treating a suicidal patient covered by a managed care system:

1. Get to know the crisis/case management/hospital admission system covering your patient. Many managed systems will have an assigned case manager for patients who have been hospitalized. If no case manager has been assigned, you may wish to request one. Establish a working relationship with this person, if possible, *before* your patient is in crisis. Find out how to alert the appropriate crisis center of an impending problem. Be available to the crisis clinician if your patient calls.
2. If you are calling a managed care system for the first time to request an admission, be aware that many systems use clerical personnel as first-line contacts. Do not hesitate, when appropriate, to ask to speak with a clinician.

3. Use the language of *medical necessity* when asking for authorization for admission. Most managed systems use a criteria set for medical necessity of admission and continued stay. While the specific criteria set may be proprietary and therefore not readily available to the clinician seeking authorization of services, the overarching principle is that treatment becomes medically necessary when lack of that treatment would be likely to result in harm to the patient. For suicidal patients, the universal considerations are dangerousness to self or others and failure of less intensive treatment settings to provide adequate protection. Explain your clinical reasoning rather than asserting your authority or saying that you "know the patient best." Be clear about the risks to the patient if the treatment is not authorized. Be clear about your treatment plan in the short-, intermediate-, and long-term and your plans for follow-up after discharge.
4. Be willing to negotiate with the case manager or reviewer. Listen with an open mind to the alternatives. There may be resources available (respite beds, day hospitals, acute residential treatment centers) that would serve as well as, or better than, a hospital, particularly if your patient is chronically and repeatedly suicidal.
5. If you disagree with the utilization manager about authorizing care that you feel is necessary, there are several options: ask for a consultation, ask for a "second level" review by a psychiatrist, ask for a forensic evaluation, or ask for an explication of the appeals process. Document your disagreement with the reviewer and your attempts to appeal. Ultimately, you, the patient, the patient's significant others, and the hospital may need to confer about whether to hospitalize without coverage (pending appeal) and bear financial risk, or not to hospitalize and bear medicolegal risk (see Chapter 8, this volume, for a fuller discussion of this issue).
6. If you feel that DBT may be helpful for your patient, discuss this with the case manager and offer to work with the managed care company to work out coding and coverage for these services. Point out that DBT is an evidence-based treatment that has been shown to reduce hospital days and that it is becoming the community standard of care for chronically suicidal patients with borderline personality disorder. As a precedent, be aware that one managed care company (Massachusetts Behavioral Health Partnership 1998) has developed specific authorization procedures and coding for DBT. A "unit" of treatment, coded as 90853D, is defined as 7 calendar days of DBT, including individual therapy (60 minutes), DBT skills group (120–135 minutes), telephone

consultation (15 minutes), and a consultation team meeting (60 minutes). Up to four units are authorized at a time. Reauthorization is dependent on the use of a standardized assessment instrument.

Conclusion

The major tasks in suicide crisis management are to provide access to care, assess suicide risk, provide immediate intervention, and lay the groundwork for future treatment. Managed systems offer advantages of coordination, consultation, clinical guidelines, and a full spectrum of services, but these systems run the risk of undertreatment. A crucial element in assessment is distinguishing between acute lethality and the chronic suicidal and self-harm behavior of some patients with personality disorders. Too often, long-term growth of such individuals is impeded by the regression caused by unnecessary hospitalization for self-injurious behavior. Managed psychiatric emergency services with holding bed capacity may increase their effectiveness by implementing a screening and intervention process that draws on cognitive behavioral and/or dialectical behavior therapy theory and techniques. Such a service, supported by appropriate medical and psychiatric evaluation and disposition options, provides appropriate access, guides assessment, and facilitates disposition decisions. The acute intervention, following assessment of immediate risk, uses cognitive behavioral, skill-based approaches to help the patient acquire skills for appropriate self-management to lay the groundwork for longer-term growth and prevention of future crises.

References

Bassuk E, Gerson S: Chronic crisis patients: a discrete group. Am J Psychiatry 137:1513–1517, 1980

Beautrais AL, Joyce PR, Mulder RT, et al: Prevalence and comorbidity of mental disorders in patients making serious suicide attempts: a case-control study. Am J Psychiatry 153:1009–1014, 1996

Beck AT, Brown G, Berchick RJ, et al: Relationship between hopelessness and ultimate suicide: a replication with psychiatric outpatients. Am J Psychiatry 147:190–195, 1990

Ellison JM, Blum N, Barsky AJ: Repeat visitors in the psychiatric emergency service: a critical review of the data. Hospital and Community Psychiatry 37:37–41, 1986

Ennis J, Barnes R, Spenser H: Management of the repeatedly suicidal patient. Can J Psychiatry 30:535–538, 1985

Fawcett J, Clark DC, Busch KA: Assessing and treating the patient at risk for suicide. Psychiatric Annals 23:244–255, 1993

Harvard Pilgrim Health Care: Patient Assessment Tool. Boston, MA, Harvard Pilgrim Health Care, 1996

Isometsa ET, Henriksson MM, Heinekkinen ME, et al: Suicide among subjects with personality disorders. Am J Psychiatry 153:667–673, 1996

Jacobs D: Evaluation and care of suicidal behavior in emergency settings. Int J Psychiatry Med 12:295–310, 1982

Kirstein L, Prusoff B, Weissman MM, et al: Utilization review of treatment for suicide attempters. Am J Psychiatry 132:22–27, 1975

Kreitman N: Age and parasuicide ('attempted suicide'). Psychol Med 6:113–121, 1976

Lazarus A: Managed competition and access to emergency psychiatric care. Hospital and Community Psychiatry 44:1134–1141, 1993

Lester D: The effectiveness of suicide prevention centers. Suicide Life Threat Behav 23:263–267, 1993

Linehan MM: Dialectical behavior therapy: a cognitive behavioral approach to parasuicide. Journal of Personality Disorders 1:328–333, 1987

Linehan MM: Cognitive-Behavioral Treatment of Borderline Personality Disorder. New York, Guilford, 1993a

Linehan MM: Workbook for the Cognitive-Behavioral Treatment of Borderline Personality Disorder. New York, Guilford, 1993b

Linehan MM: Behavioral treatments of suicidal behaviors. Ann N Y Acad Sci 836:302–328, 1997

Linehan MM, Armstrong HE, Suarez A, et al: Cognitive-behavioral treatment of chronically parasuicidal borderline patients. Arch Gen Psychiatry 48:1060–1065, 1991

Linehan MM, Heard HL, Armstrong HE: Naturalistic follow-up of a behavioral treatment for chronically parasuicidal borderline patients. Arch Gen Psychiatry 50:971–974, 1993

Lurie L, Moscovice IS, Finch M, et al: Does capitation affect the health of the chronically mentally ill? Results from a randomized trial. JAMA 267:3300–3304, 1992

Maltsberger JT: Calculated risks in the treatment of intractably suicidal patients. Psychiatry 57:199–212, 1994

Massachusetts Behavioral Health Partnership: New outpatient benefit: dialectical behavior therapy. Clinical Alert 2(9):1–3, 1998

McNiel DE, Binder RL: The impact of hospitalization on clinical assessment of suicide risk. Psychiatr Serv 48:204–208, 1997

Morgan HG, Jones EM, Owen JH: Secondary prevention of non-fatal deliberate self-harm. The Green Card Study. Br J Psychiatry 163:111–112, 1993

Reinecke M: Suicide and depression, in Cognitive Behavioral Strategies in Crisis Management. Edited by Dattilio M, Freeman A. New York, Guilford, 1994, pp 67–103

Risk Management Foundation of Harvard Medical Institutions: Guidelines for Identification, Assessment and Treatment Planning for Suicidality. Cambridge, MA, Harvard Medical Institutions, Risk Management Foundation, 1996

Rissmiller DJ, Steer R, Ranieri WF, et al: Factors complicating cost containment in the treatment of suicidal patients. Hospital and Community Psychiatry 45:782–788, 1994

Roy A: Risk factors for suicide in psychiatric patients. Arch Gen Psychiatry 39:1089–1095, 1982

Sabin JE: A credo for ethical managed care in mental health practice. Hospital and Community Psychiatry 45:859–860, 1994

Segal SP, Watson M, Goldfinger S, et al: Civil commitment in the emergency room. Arch Gen Psychiatry 45:748–761, 1988

Stanford EJ, Goetz RR, Bloom JD: The no harm contract in the emergency assessment of suicidal risk. J Clin Psychiatry 55:344–348, 1994

van der Sande R, Buskins E, Allart E, et al: Psychosocial intervention following suicide attempt: a systematic review of treatment interventions. Acta Psychiatr Scand 96:43–50, 1997

CHAPTER 3

Managed Care, Brief Hospitalization, and Alternatives to Hospitalization in the Care of Suicidal Patients

Patricia A. Harney, Ph.D.

Clinicians[1] in outpatient and emergency settings worry increasingly, in the current health care climate, about the availability of safe and meaningful care options for suicidal patients. As hospital stays shorten, under the watchful eyes of managed care reviewers or administrators of capitated contracts, patients and clinicians feel growing pressure to accomplish ever more given ever fewer days. Opportunities for trimming services and cutting costs in outpatient care, too, have attracted the attention of managed systems, so that outpatient clinicians can no longer take for

---

[1]The focus of this chapter, alternatives to hospitalization, requires discussion of treatment sites that are staffed primarily by nonpsychiatrist mental health professionals. The generic term *clinician* will be used, therefore, with clarification when discipline-specific tasks such as prescribing are discussed.

granted the authorization of a number of sessions sufficient for initiating, undertaking, and completing a treatment at the pace that might seem most appropriate.

The spread of managed care, while limiting access to both inpatient and outpatient services, has paradoxically provided fertile soil for the growth of clinical programs with an intensity of care intermediate between inpatient and outpatient. In some geographical areas, the continuum of potential clinical services now includes a "continuous care" spectrum that includes partial hospitalization programs, acute residential treatment placements, 24-hour "observation" beds, and home-based services. Clinicians who work in such settings[2] struggle to reconcile two opposing forces: the pressure to lower costs by limiting the use of clinical services and the pressure to make use of the broadened range of options to provide quality care and promote risk management. This chapter is intended as a guide for clinicians who have access to different levels of care, to increase their familiarity with the processes of triage, acute care evaluation with focal treatment planning, brief hospitalization, and choice of alternatives to hospitalization.

When Is Outpatient Care Too Little Care?

Outpatient therapists who treat suicidal patients often feel vulnerable and isolated in their work. The fear that a patient in our care may harm himself or herself fills us with distressing feelings about loss, death, lack of control, and fears of incompetence. Further, we live in litigious times and cannot help but worry that our patient's death will be accompanied by serious legal consequences even when appropriate care was rendered. The availability of emergency services and inpatient units for backup to outpatient clinicians who treat patients at high risk for suicide has long been an important source of support for therapists who are engaged in this type of work.

Under current managed systems' influence, a patient's suicidal risk must be imminent in order to justify authorization of intensive services such as hospitalization. Therapists may not want to refer a patient for hospitalization when they cannot be sure that the patient will be hospitalized. Patients

---

[2] The issues faced by clinicians in areas that have not yet developed continuous care systems are worthy of a separate paper and beyond the scope of the present chapter; however, the reader is referred to Chapter 2 and Appendix B of this book for preliminary suggestions.

might seem too vulnerable to go through an evaluation with an unfamiliar clinician, especially one that would require a lengthy wait in an emergency room, only to be followed by a denial of the services recommended by their outpatient therapist. If the patient went to the emergency room only reluctantly or involuntarily, such an outcome could damage a fragile therapeutic alliance. If the emergency room clinician and/or the insurer deny acute care services, the patient may return to outpatient treatment with a damaged alliance with his or her therapist.

To function effectively under such circumstances, clinicians need to be knowledgeable about not only the assessment of suicide risk but also the appropriate emergency triage process for each patient. This task might seem overwhelming. Clinicians should remember, however, that the patient is probably more overwhelmed by his or her crisis situation than the clinician is by insurance regulations. Clinicians need to think carefully about how to discuss the need for an acute care assessment with a patient. One should not make definitive statements such as "You need to be in the hospital," even though the therapist should be prepared to appeal a denial of services that seems unwarranted. Finally, clinicians must take care to communicate effectively with emergency room clinicians. Because patients may communicate only partial information to an emergency room clinician, outpatient clinicians should communicate as much appropriate information as possible to the emergency room staff in order to ensure the most comprehensive assessment and to make clear the reasons for and goals of hospitalization. The presence of acute and serious danger typically confers on the therapist the right to convey such information, but whenever possible the clinician should acknowledge the treatment alliance by obtaining the patient's informed consent for such communications.

Triage in Managed Systems

Health plans vary greatly in their emergency triage protocols. Indemnity insurance covers medically necessary care in any emergency room. Some managed health plans, on the other hand, designate specific facilities as the only acceptable ones for dispensing services or evaluating patients for hospitalization. Other managed plans may employ a crisis or "screening" team that will travel to emergency rooms in different geographical locations to assess patients on site.

Some health plans have such specific requirements that the outpatient therapist needs to make several calls and the patient must speak with several different clinicians prior to obtaining approval for an inpatient admission. In one clinician's experience, for example, a suicidal patient was required by her health maintenance organization (HMO) first to see her primary care physician for medical clearance, then to travel to a designated emergency room, where a mobile crisis team employed by the HMO would meet her. The outpatient therapist therefore spoke with three separate professionals in the midst of this patient's suicidal crisis: the primary care physician, the triage nurse in the designated emergency room, and the HMO crisis clinician. Not surprisingly, the patient found it difficult to navigate this system alone. Needless to say, the therapist also donated several unreimbursed hours of extra clinical work that required rescheduling of other patients.

Sometimes, in a crisis of ambiguous severity, the safest course of action is to send the patient to the nearest emergency room even without assurance that there will be reimbursement for services by the insurer. When a patient is in a particularly vulnerable state and is seen by the therapist as being at very high risk to harm himself or herself, the therapist may decide that the process of informing the patient of the requirements of his or her health plan may increase the patient's anxiety in a potentially dangerous way. If, for instance, the patient has already harmed himself or herself, he or she should be evaluated medically as quickly as possible. If the patient refuses outright to seek additional assistance and is, in the clinician's view, clearly at significant risk for suicide, the clinician should involve the police or an ambulance for escort to the nearest emergency room. Clinicians should know that police departments vary in their willingness to involuntarily detain and transport a patient to an emergency room. Psychiatrists in many jurisdictions have the authority to enlist police aid in involuntary commitment of a patient, while nonmedical mental health clinicians may need to involve the patient's psychiatrist or primary care physician to initiate this process.

The risk that a suicidal patient will harm himself or herself may increase during the time it takes to navigate a triage system to obtain emergency services complicated by managed care gatekeepers. Access problems, for example, were cited as one source of the 7% higher attempted suicide rate found in a capitated plan compared with a fee-for-service plan (Lurie et al. 1992).[3] Clinicians should not, therefore, delay necessary crisis treatment because of insurance questions. Rather, it is most appropriate to find the immediate ser-

---

[3]The possibly contrasting finding of no increase in suicides within one managed care plan, as noted in Chapter 2 of this book, may be explained by that specific plan's attention to access and the ready availability to its members of acute care.

vices needed, even if this must involve a nondesignated facility, and to document the reasons for doing so in sufficient detail so that the patient may later be able to appeal for reimbursement on the basis of the acute medical necessity of the treatment.

Therapists should communicate with the clinicians in the emergency room in any way possible. Sending a patient over to the emergency room without communicating the clinical information held by the outpatient therapist compromises the assessment that takes place. Clinicians should communicate succinctly, focusing on information that is directly relevant to the patient's risk status. This information should include both the general demographic factors that are known to be associated with suicide (see Chapter 1, this volume) and the specific psychodynamic and diagnostic factors that are relevant to the individual patient's risk.

What options are available to outpatient clinicians when they feel strongly that their patients are at high risk for self- or other harm, when they feel they cannot safely treat a patient on an outpatient basis without additional backup, and when the insurer denies authorization for an inpatient admission? The outpatient clinician can (and actually must!) advocate for additional care in a number of ways. First, he or she should consult with the patient's other mental health care providers—for example a prescribing psychiatrist or nurse clinical specialist—to coordinate the effort to increase the intensity of a patient's care. Next, the primary care physician should become involved, since he or she may have additional information about the patient that could assist the clinician in either doing the outpatient work or making a formal appeal of the denied authorization. Collateral informants are important sources of information in any crisis and are crucial in the care of treatment of children or adolescents. With young patients, the outpatient clinician should gather clinical data routinely from the patient's family, school, and any other collateral treater involved in the case. These consultations should be documented, because this information may allow the outpatient clinician to make a stronger case for an increase in services and, therefore, form the basis of an appeal. Finally, clinicians can contact the insurer directly and request an expedited response to their appeal. In some states, such as Massachusetts, legislation has been considered that requires insurers to respond to such a request with an expedited review process.

Not every patient who reports suicidal ideation will require hospitalization. For intermittently or chronically suicidal patients, the outpatient therapist may choose to work through some crises by making use of increased outpatient supports. Intermittently or chronically suicidal patients often receive services from several outpatient treaters: an individual therapist, a pharmacotherapist,[4] a primary care physician, and possibly a group therapist. For many patients with intermittent or chronic suicidal ideation, hospitalization is just one phase in a very long series of treatments. Outpatient therapists therefore must formulate appropriate treatment goals regarding suicide.

Triage-Oriented Formulation and the Value of Focal Treatment Planning

The diagnostic process in crises must include both a syndromal diagnosis (DSM Axis I and/or Axis II) and an assessment of the situational factors precipitating an acute need for care. The concept of focal treatment planning has been invoked to describe the process of treatment for acute psychiatric problems. Several elements are critical in the formulation of a focal problem (Bennett 1997; Harper 1989, 1997). Three questions constitute the primary frame of inquiry: Why now? (What brings the patient to this crisis now?), What now? (What is it that the patient is willing and able to change?), and What next? (What treatment is needed in order to assist the patient in the reduction of suicide risk?). One also needs to address the issue of context: What will enable a patient to manage feelings without acting on suicidal impulses outside of the hospital? Finally, one needs to consider the biopsychosocial factors that contribute to the current crisis. Formulating the focal problem helps to assess the level of care needed by a suicidal patient at a particular point in time. These issues will be addressed later in this chapter in the discussion of different levels of care.

---

[4]The use of this term, which is common parlance in clinical settings, does not indicate an endorsement of the narrowed role served by psychiatrists in many agencies. There is no unique credential for such a role, and serving narrowly as a "pharmacotherapist," "prescriber," or "med backup" does not excuse the psychiatrist from conducting his or her own thorough clinical assessment of each patient treated. Currently there is much controversy over whether such narrowing of the psychiatrist's role creates an unacceptable risk of treatment fragmentation, and some authorities have even questioned this approach's cost-effectiveness. Beitman (1996) and Goldman et al. (1998) are currently the most persuasive opponents of "splitting" treatment; unfortunately, their studies do not focus on suicidal patients, examine quality or outcome measures, or take into account the complexity of the treatment often required. Beitman (1996), for example, argued that a 20- to 30-minute psychotherapy/medication management visit provided by a psychiatrist is less costly than the sum of costs for a 40- to 50-minute psychotherapy visit with a nonphysician psychotherapist and a brief medication management visit with a psychiatrist. To conduct a 20- to 30-minute session with a suicidal patient in which psychotherapy and medication issues are addressed, however, seems too little time for too much work and may outweigh the risk of potential discontinuity in a treatment team approach.

Because of their frequent exposure to suicidal patients, emergency room, inpatient, or partial hospital program clinicians are particularly attuned to the gradations of suicidality and are particularly aware of the treatment decisions that must be made. Clearly, one of the largest risks is the clinician's failure to inquire about suicidality. A study of suicide assessment at a college counseling center, for instance, found that 14% of the male patients and 22% of female patients reported that they had attempted suicide in the past but that only half of these patients recalled having been asked about suicide attempts in their intake interview at the counseling center (Hahn and Marks 1996). A study by Malone et al. (1995) found a significant discrepancy between the suicide data documented in a chart review of an inpatient sample and data gathered by researchers using a semistructured suicide interview with the same patient sample. Specifically, information about the suicidality was far less often documented in the charts, even though research interviews with the same patients revealed a significant degree of suicidality among the sample. Documentation and assessment of suicidality by outpatient clinicians may be even less thorough.

Most outpatient clinicians would not (and should not) work with patients in an outpatient setting who express a clear intent to kill themselves within a specified, short-term time frame and who have a plan and means by which to kill themselves. Such patients clearly meet commitment criteria if they are unwilling to voluntarily admit themselves to a secure treatment setting. Many hospitals admit suicidal patients only when they meet these criteria. Hospitals may deny admission because insurance companies may not authorize payment for services of patients who fall short of commitment criteria. Patients who vary along any of these dimensions (intent, plan, means, and time frame) therefore create a more complex treatment dilemma for outpatient therapists. A patient who intends to kill himself or herself in the next year, for instance, or a patient with a plan and means but no imminent intent, would not be considered committable and therefore may not meet the criteria for admission to an acute or subacute facility.

What are reasonable focal problems, then, that the outpatient clinician can target for his or her work with a suicidal patient who does not meet inpatient admission criteria? An outpatient clinician might identify a focal problem with a suicidal patient as "risk of suicide as evidenced by frequent suicidal thoughts and a wish to die." Contributing factors might include biological factors such as a major depressive episode, psychological factors such as an identification with a significant person who completed suicide, and treatment factors such as unsuccessful medication trials. The focal problem should lead directly to treatment goals. Outpatient treatment for a patient with the above-described focal problem may include obtaining a psychiatric consultation to clarify diagnosis and understand the failure of the previous medication trials, and exploring in psychotherapy the identification with the deceased significant person.

The issue of "focal problems" is more complicated for the outpatient clinician than for clinicians in acute or subacute programs because of the longer-term potential of the treatment relationship. Nonetheless, this concept may be applied to outpatient work with suicidal patients. In fact, it may be the purview of outpatient clinical work, not inpatient work, to reduce the longer-term (but not acute) risk of suicide. A prospective study that examined clinicians' estimates of patients' short- and long-term suicide risk at admission and discharge found that clinicians' estimates of short-term risk, but not long-term risk, were significantly reduced over the course of a hospitalization (McNiel and Binder 1997). Continued risk and the management of risk are problems that now fall within the treatment domain of outpatient therapists. Results of this study imply, under the contemporary health care system, that resolution of the short-term risk of suicide is the work of the inpatient/subacute service and that resolution of the longer-term risk is the work of the outpatient team.

Isolation and alienation are central dynamics in the experience of the suicidal patient. One specific goal, therefore, that an outpatient therapist may assist the patient in achieving is widening the use of social supports. Suicidal patients may need to feel that they can reliably depend on their therapists, but their therapists should not be the only persons on whom the patients depend. For chronically suicidal patients, the therapist can assist the patients in identifying possible internal or external triggers for episodes in which suicidal thoughts increase in frequency. Trauma survivors, for instance, constitute a outpatient population at high risk. For this group of patients, feelings of anger, which may seem unacceptable to them, can trigger suicidal feelings. Sometimes, patients have a surge of suicidal thoughts when interacting with a particularly important person in their lives (e.g., a parent, a perpetrator of violence). The patient may have a complex and idiosyncratic relationship with the triggering stimulus, and the meaning of the stimulus should be explored in the treatment to better understand how to alter the relationship between the stimulus and the impulse to kill oneself.

Case Example

Marilyn is a 20-year-old college student who presented for psychotherapy. She met the diagnostic criteria for major depressive disorder. Since her boyfriend ended their 6-year relationship 2 months ago, Marilyn has had persistent thoughts of suicide. She saw her primary care physician soon after the breakup, and he prescribed sertraline 100 mg/day and zolpidem tartrate 5 mg at bedtime on an "as needed" basis for sleep. He then referred her for psychotherapy when her symptoms did not remit with medication.

Marilyn had made a suicide attempt in the previous year, also after her boyfriend ended the relationship. They reunited after her suicide attempt. As time elapsed since this second breakup, Marilyn became more hopeless about a potential reunion. She struggled daily with suicidal thoughts that were expressed in a passive manner. She wished, for instance, that she would be shot accidentally. On one occasion, she walked out alone at night in potentially dangerous neighborhoods. A focal problem in her outpatient psychotherapy was identified as her risk of self harm, as evidenced by wishes to die and potentially (but not actively) dangerous behavior. The termination of her relationship with her boyfriend was the context within which her suicidal feelings emerged. Contributing factors included a propensity for depression. For several weeks, outpatient treatment was therefore focused on the feelings of worthlessness and projected rage that were generated by the breakup. Marilyn also consulted a psychiatrist to review whether the sertraline prescribed by her primary care physician was optimal for her. Once she weathered this suicidal crisis and she became less focused on killing herself, Marilyn could focus on understanding the way in which the breakup shattered her self-esteem and building ways of protecting her esteem in the future.

The HMO to which Marilyn belonged authorized an initial eight visits for psychotherapy. In order to receive authorization for additional visits, the clinician was required to submit written documentation of mental status, presenting problems treatment goals, progress toward treatment goals, and rationale for continued care. Marilyn did not reveal the depth of her distress until the fourth or fifth visit. She reported that she had kept these feelings to herself until she felt that she knew the therapist "a little" and until she felt some sense of trust. In her request for additional visits, the clinician described the focal problem, the precipitating events, and her history. Although the paperwork required in submitting such reports was burdensome, the focal problem organizational framework allowed for clear communication of issues, treatment goals, and succinct updates in a manner that was consistent with each preceding report.

In summary, outpatient therapists should consider carefully when to refer suicidal patients for an evaluation of a higher level of care. The patient's intent, plan, means, and time frame are important elements in this assessment. When patients are not at imminent risk but continue to have suicidal thoughts and feelings, these concerns should take precedence in the outpatient psychotherapy. Understanding the factors that exacerbate suicidal thoughts and feelings, assisting patients in developing methods of coping with such distressing feelings, and helping the patient to decrease his or her social isolation are just some of the issues that an outpatient therapist can target in the treatment of a suicidal patient. The concept of focal treatment planning assists therapists in organizing their clinical information in a manner that expedites communication with outpatient utilization reviewers.

Brief Hospitalization

Clinicians who work on inpatient units often feel that they are required to do more work in less time with ever more fragile patients. Often they must reach a credible diagnosis and formulation, begin a medication, complete a medical assessment, and monitor changes in both mental and physical functioning in less than a week's time. Because so many patients admitted to an inpatient unit present with suicidal ideation, an inpatient clinician may have difficulty in discriminating between higher- and lower-risk patients. The large majority of suicidal patients seen by an inpatient clinician will not die by suicide. This fact, combined with the pressures to maintain brief lengths of stay, may numb inpatient clinicians to the potential risk of suicide. Clearly, there is a need for assessment tools with strong predictive validity, though these are not currently available.

Inpatient clinicians are required to conduct rapid but comprehensive assessments upon admission and to develop disposition plans as soon as they learn that a patient is on the unit's threshold. Family meetings need to be held and conferences with collateral treaters need to be coordinated in lightening speed. Unless clinicians have a structured approach to their work, they are at risk of feeling overwhelmed and working inefficiently. The greatest risk faced by inpatient clinicians is the possibility of discharging a patient too soon to a subacute or outpatient treatment setting, before resolution of imminent suicide risk has been achieved.

Under current constraints, inpatient clinicians may find that their treatment goals are often limited to arriving at a diagnosis and formulation, making minor medication adjustments, and reducing a patient's immediate or short-term risk status in order to allow the patient to continue their therapeutic work in an outpatient setting. Use of a multidisciplinary treatment team can help orient the clinical work, facilitate agreement on a suitable diagnosis, and monitor the effects of milieu and medications. Such teams offer holding environments for clinicians working under the stress of these demands. The other clinicians involved in the patient's next level of care (e.g., outpatient therapist, partial hospital therapist) are important individuals with whom to communicate. Such inpatient admissions can be conceptualized as "consultations" to outpatient treatment.

Managed care plans aim to admit suicidal patients to an inpatient psychiatry unit only when risk is both great and imminent. Some patients have made a potentially lethal attempt and express the wish to try again. Other patients may not have made an attempt but may possess the desire, means, and intent to do so and may be ready to take action within a specified, short-term time frame. In such cases, the focal problem would be framed as "High, or imminent risk of suicide as evidenced by recent suicide attempt, persistent wish to die, and plan to attempt again." In such cases, the clinician must explore the precipitant(s) to the suicide attempt. What led this patient to attempt suicide now? What life events have stressed the person beyond his or her capacity to bear psychic distress? What new-onset psychiatric or medical diagnosis may be relevant? The clinician also must address "What now?"—what in the patient's life needs to change in order for the death wish to transform into a will to live. Finally, the clinician needs to explore what the patient needs in order to maintain the change—in other words, what does the patient need in order to maintain a will to live, even during times when he or she might rather die? Under current constraints, the inpatient clinician might hope only for enough change to reduce the imminence of the patient's risk, such that the patient could be stepped down to a lower level of care.

Case Example

Janet, a 17-year-old woman, was admitted to an adolescent inpatient unit after a potentially lethal overdose. Upon admission to the inpatient unit, Janet expressed regret that her attempt was not successful. A verbally gifted former honors student whose grades had fallen dramatically over the past 6 months, Janet could say little about her thoughts, feelings, and experiences that may have preceded her attempt. She identified as the only stress the fact that her boyfriend had recently ended their relationship. Feelings of rejection were certainly prominent in her presentation. She didn't feel, however, that her disappointment at this breakup accounted fully for her despair. She denied any other life difficulties. The only clue to family dysfunction was evidenced in Janet's comments that her mother slept most of every day.

In a family meeting, Janet's mother presented as extremely depressed. Discussion in several family meetings revealed that Janet felt neglected by her mother and was unable to sustain feelings of self-worth in the course of disappointments. Over time, Janet's acute suicidality diminished as she became more aware of her desire for greater connection with her family. Early in her inpatient admission, the unit psychiatrist chose not to prescribe medication until Janet was more fully known. After a week on the unit, Janet was more forthcoming about her own depression, and a medication trial was initiated (sertraline 100 mg/day). Although her imminent risk of self-harm attenuated, she expressed great concern about her discharge and worried that "things at home would be the same." At this point, Janet was ready for a step-down to partial hospitalization, where she could take responsibility for her safety and feel assured that her parents would be required to continue to address these issues intensively.

Janet's stay on the inpatient unit and then in the partial hospital program was longer than average, and the utilization reviewer for her HMO was concerned about her potential for regression. The partial hospital clinician felt that Janet's family was not responding to treatment as quickly as she would have hoped. The clinician persuaded the reviewer that the severity of Janet's overdose, her own positive progress in treatment, and her family's very limited progress warranted a longer length of stay until more intensive supports could be identified to use following her discharge from the program. Without such supports, Janet would return to a similarly neglectful home situation that could precipitate another suicide attempt. A school counselor was then able to place Janet in a therapeutic program within her school district that modeled some of the features of the partial hospital program. Thus, a more structured and supportive school environment might compensate partially for the family's slow progress.

Partial Hospitalization

The partial hospital clinician's role may be the most complex in the continuous care system. When patients are referred from inpatient units, the partial hospital clinician must gather information from that admission as well as from the outpatient clinician. Overall coordination of care following discharge from the partial hospital program often falls to the partial hospital clinician, who must integrate information obtained from outpatient treaters with information obtained from the inpatient clinicians in order to facilitate the best discharge and aftercare plan.

Partial hospital patients are often in a fragile state. Even though they may not be imminently suicidal, they may be still be on the brink of serious self-harm. Careful work is therefore required to ensure a patient's safety after hours and on weekends. Further, the partial hospital milieu is often less intensively supervised than the inpatient milieu. The potential anxiety felt by the partial hospital clinician may be greater than that experienced by inpatient clinicians, because the partial hospital clinician does not have the assurance afforded other clinicians by the 24-hour surveillance.

Advantages to the partial hospital clinician are that partial hospital admissions may be somewhat longer than inpatient stays and therefore may allow for greater opportunity to understand better the dynamic factors that contributed to the crisis. This understanding can then be used to reduce suicide risk.

Case Example

Renee is a 16-year-old girl who had been in outpatient psychotherapy with the same therapist on a weekly basis for about 9 months. She had been in psychotherapy in the past, at ages 12, 14, and 15, with several different therapists, but after a period of time she typically refused treatment. Her parents rarely followed through with recommendations for family treatment. Nine months was the longest period of time that Renee ever worked with a therapist.

Renee was initially seen for a crisis evaluation when she was 12 years old and then a number of times intermittently. Her health plan's capitated contract designated a specific hospital for Renee's assessment and care, and each time Renee entered a crisis, she was seen at that same facility. The hospital maintained a small team of clinicians to meet with patients in crisis who were part of the capitated population. On this team, Renee was assigned a particular clinician, so that each time she was evaluated in crisis, she was evaluated by the same clinician. Although Renee refused to meet with her outpatient therapist, she developed a working alliance with her crisis clinician, who in turn developed a good relationship with Renee's parents. The crisis clinician, then, was able to develop a formulation with which to understand Renee's frequent crises.

Her parents felt controlled by her emotional outbursts, and they frequently requested hospitalization for her. She had been diagnosed with attention-deficit disorder at age 12 and was seen every few months by a psychiatrist who prescribed methylphenidate 10 mg bid. By age 15, she had also been diagnosed with bipolar II disorder and was prescribed divalproex 1,500 mg/day. She was extremely argumentative with authority figures and often threatened to kill other people, although she had never been physically aggressive. On one occasion, at age 13, she carved her favorite rock singer's name into her leg. Her parents were concerned about this self-destructive behavior and again requested hospitalization. In a crisis evaluation, Renee denied any self-destructive intent when she cut herself. Once again, outpatient treatment was recommended but not followed.

When Renee turned 16, her psychiatrist suggested psychotherapy during a period of relative stability. This marked the first time that Renee entered psychotherapy during a period of calm rather than of crisis. Renee was offered a choice of therapists in the outpatient department of the hospital where her psychiatrist worked. Renee actually had the option to meet for psychotherapy with the crisis clinician she had worked with in the other capacity for several years. For the first time, Renee enjoyed meeting with a therapist, and over time she began to assume more responsibility for her self-control. She demonstrated considerable insight, commenting at times about her desire for attention and her feeling that she would receive attention only if she were loud and disruptive. After a period of time, Renee missed several psychotherapy sessions. Both her mother and the therapist were lax in rescheduling appointments, and eventually a month passed from the last time Renee was seen.

Renee's therapist received a call one night from Renee's mother, who reported that Renee had overdosed on more than 20 pills and was in the emergency room. The therapist consulted with the emergency room clinician. During the crisis evaluation, Renee admitted that she had tried to kill herself but felt sick and foolish afterward, and she felt convinced that she would not attempt to kill herself again. At the end of the evaluation, the emergency room clinician and the managed care reviewer recommended an admission to a partial hospital program.

During her partial hospital admission, clinicians helped Renee focus on understanding what went wrong. After a period of relative stability and no history of suicide attempts, her current overdose was difficult to understand. Renee commented that she had been feeling pretty well until her boyfriend broke up with her. This breakup occurred at the same time her best friend attempted suicide and was being treated on an inpatient unit where Renee's therapist worked. After several days in her partial program, Renee admitted that she felt that no one was paying attention to her and that she was jealous of the attention her friend was receiving. The fact that her mother and therapist let appointments go by without being rescheduled because Renee was stable led her to feel as if she needed to "take serious action" in order to be cared for. Once Renee was reconnected with her therapist and they discussed these issues, Renee could be safely discharged from her partial hospital program. She continued to remain stable in weekly outpatient treatment and to develop ways of communicating her needs in a more proactive manner.

Renee's partial hospital admission was brief, focused, and led to a positive outcome. Her admission to that level of care, as opposed to an inpatient level of care, may surprise some because of the severity of her overdose. Her therapist's involvement in the crisis evaluation allowed for critical information to be considered: that Renee had never attempted suicide in the past, that Renee had previously identified that her disruptive behavior was often connected to a wish for attention, and that she had been doing well in psychotherapy before she dropped out of treatment. Timely communication between the outpatient therapist and the crisis clinician assisted in identifying the appropriate level of care and the focal problem for treatment. Renee's case also attests to the need for longer-term, outpatient psychotherapy for patients who are at risk for self-destructive behavior and for utilizing higher levels of care.

Renee's case involved the use of a range of services within one facility: outpatient, inpatient, partial hospital, and crisis intervention. Her case illustrates some advantages of a capitated system that relies on the use of a designated facility. There was continuity of care in her relationships with clinicians over the course of several years and across different levels of care. The formulation that evolved over many clinical encounters led to an accurate assessment of Renee's need for partial hospital treatment during the most recent crisis. (Clinicians who did not know Renee may have recommended a higher level of care after her overdose.)

There are also disadvantages to using a designated facility, however. If clinicians in one facility develop a shared formulation of a patient, they may miss important information that might have been detected by a consultant outside the facility. In addition, the designated facility system restricts patient choice. Patients who are dissatisfied with the care they receive at a designated facility may face a lengthy process to get approval for care elsewhere. Or, they may be asked to change treaters outside the mental health system (e.g., a primary care physician) in order to affiliate with their preferred designated facility in order to receive mental health care.

Acute Residential Treatment

Acute residential treatment involves 24-hour care that typically is not contained within a locked facility. The availability of psychiatric and nursing staff varies, and staffing is leaner than on an inpatient unit. Patients admitted to acute residential settings must maintain responsibility for their safety because of the relatively lower degree of clinical supervision available. Acute residential programs are maintained either in the community as free-standing agencies or in affiliation with hospitals as part of a broader continuum of care. Reimbursement for this level of care remains variable, and a number of insurers do not pay for acute residential treatment.

Acute residential treatment units were developed for patients who may be at acute risk of self or other harm if they continue to live in their current situation. Acute residential settings provide containment and an environmental intervention in a less costly manner than an inpatient admission. Clinicians typically work with patients in order to step down quickly to a partial hospital level of care. In the case of some children and adolescents, stability that is achieved only at this level of care may suggest the need for a longer-term placement in a residential school.

A study by Sledge and colleagues (1996a) compared the efficacy of day treatment with a residential component and inpatient treatment on the symptoms and psychiatric functioning of patients in need of acute psychiatric treatment. Only patients who required one-on-one supervision in the first day of treatment, those who were intoxicated, and those who required 24-hour medical attention were excluded from the study. In a randomized design, patients were assigned either to an inpatient program or to the day treatment with residential services. No differences in outcome were found. Treatment offered in both settings appeared equally effective in reducing psychiatric symptoms and in improved functioning. In addition, the investigators compared the costs of both programs (Sledge et al. 1996b). Inpatient treatment costs approximately 20% more to deliver services than day treatment with residential service. Cost savings of the day treatment/residential service was especially high for patients with affective disorders. Costs to operate the inpatient program were significantly greater than costs to operate the day treatment/residential program. The direct service costs of the two programs were similar.

Another study that compared acute residential treatment and inpatient treatment also found that both programs succeeded in reducing psychiatric symptoms but that the average length of stay in the acute residential program was greater than in the inpatient program (Fenton et al. 1998).

Case Example

Don is a 26-year-old man who had been diagnosed with bipolar mood disorder at the age of 19. During his depressive episodes, he hears hallucinations commanding him to commit suicide. He was first hospitalized at age 19 following a serious suicide attempt. With medication (most recently divalproex 500 mg tid and risperidone 2 mg bid) and outpatient psychotherapy, he has been able to complete a bachelor's degree while living at home with his mother.

Several events have precipitated relapse over the years. Early in the course of his illness, Don was intermittently compliant with his medication. Noncompliance typically resulted in relapse and eventual hospitalization. In the last few years, Don has developed a greater understanding of his illness and manages his medications well. External stressors, however, sometimes precipitate an exacerbation of depressive symptoms and suicidal ideation.

Don's therapist referred him for an emergency psychiatric evaluation when his mother was near death from cancer. Don was well known to the emergency screening team at this time. Although his therapist made the referral, Don wanted assistance, knowing that his mother's death would disrupt much of the stability he had achieved. He would require significant support to cope with the immediate loss, as well as support to adjust to the differences he would experience in his life without his mother's presence. His suicidal preoccupations revolved around the notion that he would join her in death. He had demonstrated a good ability to make use of therapeutic support, however. Although he was at some risk of suicide given his history and current status, the emergency room screening clinician recommended an admission to an acute residential program in order to offer Don the containment and support he needed while reinforcing his ability to maintain some independence. During his 2-week admission, Don received support through his mother's death and funeral service and obtained assistance in implementing an alternative living plan so that he did not return to his home alone. Support and assistance in creating a new living situation constituted the focal problems of his admission.

Economic factors have encouraged the development of acute residential programs. In addition to potentially providing a cost-effective alternative to inpatient care, such programs offer a liberating alternative for patients with long histories of repeated hospitalization who may feel that a readmission to an inpatient unit would constitute failure. Don viewed his admission to the acute residential program as a temporary respite rather than a repetition of inpatient care that he had received many times in the past.

Observation/Holding Beds

Observations beds, also referred to as holding beds or 24-hour beds, serve a number of purposes in providing alternatives to hospitalization. They allow clinicians to evaluate an at-risk patient for an extended period of time in order to determine whether an inpatient admission is necessary. They also offer temporary respite to patients who regress quickly during an inpatient or partial hospital admission. Patients who require alternative home placements can be admitted to an observation bed while clinicians coordinate the necessary disposition.

One study investigated whether the use of observation beds actually diverts inpatient admissions (Gillig et al. 1989). In this study, inpatient admissions at two psychiatric units at different medical centers were compared. One had the capacity to hold patients for 24 hours before deciding disposition; the other did not. Results revealed that the emergency service with an observation bed capacity had lower hospitalization rates (36%) than the unit without this capacity (52%). Of the patients admitted to an observation bed, 46% were admitted to an inpatient unit, and 50% returned home. The remaining patients were referred to a supervised group home. Of the patients who were not admitted to the inpatient setting after placement on the observation bed, 7.5% were hospitalized within the next 30 days. Clinicians in the study cited the ability to assess suicide potential as the most common reason for using the 24-hour bed. Other less commonly cited reasons included assessing dangerousness to others, gathering additional history, ensuring medical stability, and linking with alternative placements.

Case Example

Sarah is a 20-year-old woman who lives with her parents while she attends a local college. She has met the criteria for major depressive disorder of moderate severity with recurrent episodes. During her late adolescence, she made potentially lethal suicide attempts on two separate occasions. After each attempt, she was admitted to an inpatient unit. Outpatient psychotherapy had helped her develop an understanding of her suicidal impulses, which included a recognition of the self-punitive, masochistic introjects that supported her suicidality. She experienced a reduction in the frequency of her suicidal ideation over the course of her 2-year psychotherapy, and she developed ways of soothing herself that were not self-punitive.

In the context of anticipating her therapists' extended vacation, however, Sarah became increasingly depressed and suicidal. She kept these feelings to herself until the week before her therapist's leave. The therapist was understandably worried and wanted to make sure that Sarah's safety was addressed. In the session prior to the therapist's leave, Sarah was unable to discuss the meaning of these feelings and potential ways of coping with them. The therapist was so concerned that she recommended an evaluation for an inpatient admission. Although Sarah agreed to the evaluation, she was vehemently opposed to a readmission. Her past history and the intensity of her current despair, however, concerned the evaluating clinician. The managed care utilization reviewer recommended an overnight admission, to which Sarah, the evaluating clinician, and her therapist agreed.

Sarah took the admission as an opportunity to discuss her anger toward her therapist, and she began to examine the way in which aggression, in addition to self-punishment, was related to her suicidal thoughts. She also had the opportunity to participate in developing an alternative disposition. Sarah's awakening insight to another aspect of her internal dynamics and her participation in this planning demonstrated her ability to take responsibility for her safety. Her participation in planning the alternative disposition also increased her compliance, which might not have developed if she had been hospitalized against her will.

Conclusion

Over the past two decades, the care of suicidal patients has been significantly altered by the pressure to decrease or divert inpatient psychiatric admissions. Such changes have the potential to benefit or harm the patients involved. The burdens on clinicians who care for these patients in all levels of care have increased. Patients sometimes get caught in the crossfire between clinicians' frustrations with the managed mental health care system and their desire to deliver adequate care.

A number of alternatives to inpatient hospitalization have been developed in an attempt to reduce or divert inpatient psychiatric admissions. Accessing these systems during a patient's suicidal crisis requires great skill, preparation, and knowledge on the part of the clinician. The treatment alternatives have the potential benefits of reducing unnecessary restrictions on the part of patients and allowing patients greater autonomy in their care. Treatment alternatives are often cost-effective as well. At the same time, a complex, continuous care system, with many points of communication involving many more professionals than ever before, creates opportunities for communication breakdown and time delay. Unfortunately, such breakdowns and time delays can result in the suicidal patient's acting out his or her impulses. Clinicians, managed health care administrators, and policymakers need to continue to review this system so that patient care remains the primary objective.

References

Beitman BD: Integrating pharmacotherapy and psychotherapy: an emerging field of study. Bull Menninger Clin 60:160–173, 1996

Bennett MJ: Focal psychotherapy, in Acute Care Psychiatry: Diagnosis and Treatment. Edited by Sederer L, Rothschild A. Baltimore, MD, Williams & Wilkins, 1997, pp 355–373

Fenton WS, Mosher LR, Herrell JM, et al: Randomized trial of general hospital and residential alternative care for patients with severe and persistent mental illness. Am J Psychiatry 155:516–522, 1998

Gillig PM, Hillard JR, Bell J, et al: The psychiatric emergency service holding area: effect on utilization of inpatient resources. Am J Psychiatry 146:369–372, 1989

Goldman W, McCulloch J, Cuffel B, et al: Outpatient utilization patterns of integrated and split psychotherapy and pharmacotherapy for depression. 49:477–482, 1998

Hahn WK, Marks LI: Client receptiveness to routine assessment of past suicide attempts. Professional Psychology: Research and Practice 27:592–594, 1996

Harper G: Focal inpatient treatment planning. J Am Acad Child Adolesc Psychiatry 28:31–37, 1989

Harper G: Disorders of childhood and adolescence, in Acute Care Psychiatry: Diagnosis and Treatment. Edited by Sederer L, Rothschild A. Baltimore, MD, Williams & Wilkins, 1997, pp 277–291

Lurie L, Moscovice IS, Finch M, et al. Does capitation affect the health of the chronically mentally ill? Results from a randomized trial. JAMA 267:3300–3304, 1992

Malone KM, Szanto K, Corbitt EB, et al: Clinical assessments versus research methods in the assessment of suicidal behavior. Am J Psychiatry 152:1601–1607, 1995

McNiel D, Binder RL: The impact of hospitalization on clinical assessment of suicide risk. Psychiatr Serv 48:204–208, 1997

Sledge WH, Tebes J, Rakfeldt J, et al: Day hospital/crisis respite versus inpatient care, Part I: clinical outcomes. Am J Psychiatry 153:1065–1073, 1996a

Sledge WH, Tebes J, Wolff N, et al: Day hospital/crisis respite care versus inpatient care, Part II: service utilization and costs. Am J Psychiatry 153:1074–1083, 1996b

CHAPTER 4

Suicidal Adolescents in Managed Care

Alan Lipschitz, M.D.

The managed care revolution is imposing new models for adolescent treatment at a time when teenage suicide remains a major public health problem. Suicide is the third leading cause of death among adolescents, after automobile accidents and homicides (National Center for Health Statistics 1994). It is an especially serious problem for adolescent boys, who commit suicide nearly five times more frequently than girls.

Suicide rates in the United States are low during childhood, rise sharply at puberty, and rise still higher in the elderly (Bell and Clark 1998; Hendin 1995). Teenagers account for 14% of the U.S. population and 16% of the suicides (Bell and Clark 1998; Hendin 1995). Among adolescents, suicide attempts are far more frequent than completed suicides, and 80% of all self-inflicted injuries occur in adolescents between the ages of 15 and 19 (Centers for Disease Control 1991, 1996; Guyer et al. 1989; Pfeffer et al. 1986).

Nearly 10% of all adolescents report attempting suicide at some time. The more serious suicide attempts occur less frequently: 5% of adolescents are injured in their suicide attempt, and about one-third of those individuals seek medical attention for the injury (Bell and Clark 1998; Centers for Disease Control 1996). Thoughts of suicide are even more common: nearly a quarter of the high school students surveyed reported that they had thought seriously about suicide during the previous year, and 20% had formulated a suicide plan (Bell and Clark 1998; Centers for Disease Control 1996).

The adolescent suicide rate began to climb in 1956, plateauing in 1994 with a peak prevalence of 32 suicides per 100,000 male youths 20 years of age. However, among black male adolescents, the suicide rate continues an alarming rise. Historically, black adolescents had lower suicide rates than whites, but from 1980 to 1995 the suicide rate for black adolescents ages 10 to 19 years more than doubled, from 2.1 to 4.5 per 100,000. During these years, suicide became more frequent among all American teenagers, but its disproportionate rise in black teenagers narrowed the black-white gap as the rate among black teenagers rose from 40% to 70% of the white teenagers' rate. This effect was most pronounced among black male adolescents in the 15- to 19-year-old cohort: their suicide rate increased 146%, compared with the 22% rise for white males in this age group (Centers for Disease Control 1998). This rising rate of suicide among black male teenagers has been attributed to social stresses or death certificate inaccuracies, but a more complex explanation is certainly necessary, since the suicide rate among black female adolescents changed little over these same years (Bell and Clark 1998).

Evaluating the Suicidal Adolescent

In all age groups, suicidal thoughts and attempts are among the strongest predictors of suicide completion. Suicidal thoughts and attempts occur so frequently in adolescents that these are only weak predictors of suicide in this age group, so determining an adolescent's suicide risk requires an individualized assessment of the adolescent's risk factors, stressors, and feelings about suicide (Restifo and Shaffer 1997). Other factors may raise the adolescent's suicide risk.

Substance Abuse Disorders and Other Psychiatric Illnesses

Psychiatric autopsy studies find that 95% of the adults who commit suicide had a substance abuse problem or other psychiatric illness. Studies find comparable prevalences in cases of adolescent suicide, with major depression and impulsive behaviors the most common psychiatric findings (Brent et al. 1993; Fowler et al. 1986; Rich et al. 1990; Shaffer et al. 1996b).

In one psychiatric autopsy study of teenagers who commited suicide, substance abuse increased the odds of suicide nearly sixfold, making it the third strongest risk factor (behind "previous suicide attempt" and "depression"). Studies find that 30%–60% of adolescents who commit suicide abused drugs or alcohol (Clark 1993; Shaffer et al. 1996b). Some studies have even suggested that the increase in adolescent alcohol use over the last 30 years is responsible for the parallel rise in adolescent suicide (Brent et al. 1987).

Psychodynamic Factors

Clinical evidence offers no support for broadly attributing all suicides to abandonment by a loved object or to inward deflection of murderous impulses. However, when these dynamics can be identified in individual cases, they serve as important foci for psychotherapeutic efforts. Modern studies find that many adolescent and adult suicide attempters cherish similar fantasies: that suicide enables reunion with a lost loved-one, or provides revenge on one's critics, or offers rebirth as a new person, cleansed of one's sins, entering a world free of the old frustrations (Hendin 1991).

Family Factors

Suicide is much more frequent in certain families. Studies on twins unequivocally demonstrate a genetic predisposition to suicide, but the increased frequency of suicide in certain families is likely to be multifactorial. Family chaos during childhood, poor communication with parents, and conflicts with family members also raise the suicide risk for adolescents. Family histories of mood disorder, aggressive conduct, and substance abuse have also been associated with an increase in adolescent suicide attempts. It is not yet clear whether the vector transmitting suicide through a family from generation to generation is a genetic predisposition, concomitant high-risk Axis I and Axis II psychiatric diagnoses, disruptions in the early childhood environment and parent-child relationships, or a combination of all these influences (Bell and Clark 1998; Greenhill and Waslick 1997).

In the United States, adolescence is a time when most people separate from their families and forge their own ways in the world. The loss of the family's support and the challenge to succeed as an independent adult can be stressful for even highly capable adolescents (Lipschitz 1990).

Gun Access

Firearms are the suicide method used most often by adolescents and adults in the United States. The presence of a gun in the home increases the risk of suicide, regardless of whether it is a long gun or a handgun, locked away or kept accessible. A gun in the home is far more likely to be used for suicide than for self-defense (Brent et al. 1987).

Acute Precipitants

The most common stressors precipitating adolescents' suicides are episodes of humiliation, discipline for misdeeds, arguments, or the loss of romantic relationships (Gould et al. 1996; Shaffer et al. 1988). Hopelessness is a strong risk factor for suicide, independent of its association with depression. Other intense and intolerable emotional states—anxiety, anger, despair—have been reported to occur immediately before and during suicide (Greenhill and Waslick 1997; Hendin 1995).

Imitation

Adolescents are particularly susceptible to suicide imitation or "contagion": committing or attempting suicide after exposure to suicidal behavior or suicide. Contact with family members who die by suicide is a risk factor for committing suicide, but the risk extends to people outside the family, and clusters of imitative suicides have followed newspaper and television reports of a suicide in the community. This "contagion" phenomenon is especially strong in adolescents who are exposed to news reports that foster imitative suicide, and the Centers for Disease Control has issued recommendations for structuring news reports to reduce the risk of contagion (Centers for Disease Control 1994).

Speeding Patient Evaluations

Assessing the forces driving adolescents to suicide, planning their treatment, and managing their care require integrating these risk factors in a comprehensive, individualized evaluation. The warning in Chapter 1 of this volume—that the need for thorough assessment can conflict with managed care pressures to shorten treatments—is of special importance with adolescents, where alliance formation and the need to obtain information from collateral informants are critically important (King 1995).

Suicidal patients tax a hospital's ability to provide prompt assessment, treatment, and discharge planning. Shortened inpatient stays pressure hospital staff members to gather data quickly from patients, their families, and their current and previous therapists in order to promptly construct a formulation of the patient's predisposition and the stressors that precipitated the suicide threat or attempt that led to admission. The acceleration of this assessment and treatment process stimulated by managed care especially burdens the staff of inpatient units where children and adolescents are treated, since these patients formerly received the most extended evaluations and the longest hospital stays.[1]

Most patients admitted to psychiatric hospitals initially improve in the hospital's structured milieu, bolstered by its empathic support, warmth, and respite from family and outside stressors. These "nonspecific therapeutic factors" help restore the patients' morale and counter suicidal patients' desperate sense that suicide offers the only possible relief from their troubles. Making explicit these nonspecific factors that improve the patient's health is precisely the art of inpatient psychiatry. Formerly, the clinician's understanding of the patient slowly unfolded over the weeks or months of an extended hospital stay; now, abbreviated stays make the therapist responsible for a more vigorous, active evaluation of the issues troubling a patient, so that prompt interventions can target the patient's specific problems. The patient's therapy must uncover and change the stressful factors in his or her life, if recovery is to be sustained outside the hospital's protective setting.

Suicidal patients are the patients most jeopardized by premature discharge from hospitals that do not fulfill their responsibility to ensure that staff in the ward or emergency room promptly gather, organize, and use the necessary data to formulate a thorough evaluation and provide individualized treatment. Expedited evaluations and shortened stays put much pressure on the therapist who assesses the patient's suicide risk. The therapist has to be able to promptly recognize and address the patient's acute and chronic suicide risk factors: psychosis, substance abuse, impulsivity, imitation, losses, despair, and past attempts. These factors cannot be considered in isolation; the therapist must weave them into a formulation that accounts for how the patient's acute symptoms emerge from the impact of recent stressors on his or her premorbid state.

The managed care company shares with the hospital and the therapist this responsibility for prompt and thorough patient evaluation. Paralleling the hospital's monitoring of its clinical staff, the managed care company must monitor its case managers to make sure that they follow inpatient treat-

---

[1]Psychiatry residents training in 1999 refuse to believe that in 1977, during my own training, a child's parents were not re-interviewed during the first week of the child's psychiatric hospitalization and medication was deliberately withheld for 4 weeks to allow observation, the gathering of a thorough history, and an individualized comprehensive diagnostic formulation.

ments closely and frequently enough to ensure that treatment progresses productively. When oversights by the case manager and the therapist allow delays in evaluation or treatment, the managed care company must still remain responsible to continue approving whatever treatment remains necessary. Consistent delays by a hospital's staff are matters for the managed care company to review with the hospital administration. The managed care company may be tempted to disapprove tomorrow's stay because of yesterday's omission, but premature discharge cannot be a patient's punishment for institutional delays.

Evolving Treatment Models

Treating adolescent patients under managed care imposes new responsibilities on the therapist, the treating institution, and the company managing the insurance benefit. Therapists and institutions who treat patients have long been held responsible for meeting professional and legal standards, but they now face new, additional requirements. Managed care companies are responsible for meeting standards set by accrediting organizations, and increasingly their corporate clients require proof that they truly *manage* care and do not simply deny payments (i.e., proof that they direct patients to competent providers and shape patient care into effective treatment). Therapists who treat patients need to understand these responsibilities in order to minimize the stress on themselves, their patient, the patient's family, and the managed care company.

Managed care has reformed the behavioral treatment of adolescents more radically than any other branch of psychiatry. Adolescent treatment, especially adolescent inpatient treatment, has always been a prime focus for managed care's efforts to curtail inpatient stays. In the 1980's, at the dawn of the managed care era, insurers and their clients—the employers who purchase health insurance for their employees—noted that a small number of patients consumed the lion's share of the benefits they paid out, and that many of these patients were adolescents hospitalized in extended, multiyear stays in remote long-term facilities. These extended stays were used to modify teenagers' disruptive behavior patterns, to reform substance abusers, or simply to give adolescents with special needs a more responsive classroom experience than their local school districts could provide. A milieu therapy model predominated, treating patients respectfully in an environment reinforcing desirable conduct, and helping them integrate these positive values thoroughly enough to overcome temptations to relapse after return to

Suicidal Adolescents in Managed Care

home. This corrective emotional experience is no longer credible as a technique for treating adolescent psychopathology, but such an empathic, supportive, and gently corrective milieu can improve adolescent's self-image and help them accept treatment.

Into this cloistered treatment environment managed care abruptly intruded the requirement that treatment be "medically necessary." Some managed care programs imposed criteria for "medical necessity" that asserted an heroic, procedure-oriented model of inpatient treatment. They reserved hospitalization for patients on the brink of causing serious harm or for patients who required procedures too dangerous to be performed outside the hospital. Few adolescent inpatients fulfilled these novel criteria, and hospitals that specialized in extended treatments were emptied.

Responsible Care

Providers and facilities dispensing milieu treatment received fewer patient referrals, while managed care companies that simply disallowed their "unnecessary" hospital days faced high rates of relapse and rehospitalization and growing protests from their clients. These poor outcomes spurred the evolution of a new phase in managed care that emphasizes "responsible care." In this treatment model, the managed care company, the treating institution, and the treating provider are jointly responsible for providing patient treatments. This model is replacing unilateral treatment criteria and adversarial case management; instead, the managed care company collaborates with willing treatment programs and providers who internalize the clinical standards of managed care.

Case Example

When she was 13 years old, Randi began secretly making fine, shallow razor cuts on her left forearm. Initially, she experienced no intent to kill herself; however, as the months went by, she began to consider suicide more frequently. At the age of 15, she cut her neck superficially after an argument with her stepmother, and she threatened to kill herself. When she was admitted to the hospital, she bonded well with her therapist, and within a few days she said that she no longer wished to commit suicide. The chaotic relationship between her stepmother and her father, however, was expected to provoke relapse if she returned home.

Before the days of managed care, a patient like Randi would be retained in the round-the-clock treatment milieu of the acute care hospital until she improved enough to function with the support of one or two outpatient therapy sessions each week. This practice is now giving way to an earlier but more gradual step-down, as inpatients transition through less intensive "levels of care." In a typical program, patients begin to attend a "partial" or "day" hospital program for 5 hours each day, while still residing on the inpatient unit. After discharge from the inpatient unit, patients continue to attend the partial hospital program for a few weeks, then transition to a 4-hour intensive outpatient program for 3 days—or evenings—each week, until they can be managed in treatment with an individual therapist.

Formerly, a patient like Randi, if her home is not ready to receive her, would be retained in the hospital, even if her clinical condition no longer required the continuous ministrations of an acute care psychiatric hospital. While awaiting discharge, she would be sent home on passes to test the stability of her improvement. In the early days of managed care, the managed care company would simply deny approval for these days of the patient's continued stay in the hospital, and the hospital would either "eat" the cost of the additional days, bill the patient or parents or another payer, or peremptorily discharge the patient home. Rapid rehospitalization often followed these discharges, with neither the hospital nor the managed care company accepting responsibility for the poor outcome. Collaboration between the managed care company and hospital allows a different approach, where the company's case managers use frequent concurrent case reviews to ensure that the hospital staff advances the patient's discharge plan—and concurrent alternative discharge plans as well—from the time of her admission. If her home is not ready to receive her, the hospital is pressed to investigate whether some relative could take the patient temporarily, or whether the patient could be sent to live in a less costly setting, such as a group home, while her individual and family treatment continues.

Interpolating day hospital programs, group homes, and transitional living facilities as temporary waystations between the hospital stay and the outpatient treatment is a novelty for many hospitals, which formerly reserved these resources for patients who required extended stays after lengthy hospitalizations. When stays were long, patients facing discharge were especially traumatized by the losses and stresses of separation and by the need to once again evolve relationships with a new therapist and new staff. Sometimes this transition was impeded when members of the treatment staff communicated their dire conviction that life ahead in the step-down program would be relatively impoverished and bereft of the enrichments hospitals provide to patients.

Now that such transfers are commonplace, collaborating hospitals accept a responsibility to facilitate successful step-downs. Transitioning patients is easiest when inpatient programs share patient information with linked partial hospital programs and when extensive communications and good liaison cross these levels of care. In well-integrated systems, treatment programs providing different levels of care share therapists and other staff members, with the same therapist treating the patient as inpatient, day hospital patient, and outpatient. The best partial hospital programs accept patients while they still reside on the inpatient unit and allow them to increasingly attend partial hospital program groups in lieu of the therapeutic activities of their inpatient ward. Patients then gradually transition from being an inpatient to being a partial hospital program patient who sleeps at home or in a group home.

Integrating these levels of care was a cherished goal of the community psychiatry movement, but it was unattainable while hospitals narrowly focused on filling their beds and maintaining a high occupancy rate. It took the managed care revolution to convince inpatient facilities that filling beds cannot be their primary objective; in the current environment, the hospital best serves its own interests by reducing its length of stay and appropriately transitioning patients to lower levels of care. Shortening inpatient hospitalizations while maintaining or raising care quality has been the central principle of managed care, as well as its single biggest cost-reducing measure. Health insurance typically covers 30–60 days per year of inpatient psychiatric treatment. To receive patients from managed care companies, hospitals that routinely held patients for this entire period have managed to reduce their average length of stay to a week or less.

In the more evolved collaborations, the hospital is not paid a per diem rate, but receives from the managed care company a flat "case rate" for treating each inpatient. These case-rated hospitals—which receive a fixed sum to treat each patient—suffer a direct financial penalty when inpatient stays are extended. In business jargon, the inpatient hospital shifts from a "profit center" to a "cost center." These hospitals bear the responsibility for providing ready access to the lower levels of care, contracting with community facilities, day hospitals, transitional residences, drug rehabilitation programs, and other facilities to give priority to accepting discharged inpatients and patients diverted from inpatient admission by prompt enrollment in one of these less intensive levels of care. This new payment paradigm reverses the traditional role of the managed care company: it no longer polices every case to reduce overutilization, but instead audits cases to ensure treatment quality and to guard against *under*utilization.

To further this flexibility, many managed care plans allow the exchange of inpatient benefit days for days of outpatient treatment in partial hospital programs; typically each inpatient benefit day can be "flexed" for 2 days of partial hospital treatment. Shortening inpatient stays helps reserve patients' benefits to cover these less intensive treatments.

Drug Rehabilitation

Managed care has similarly shortened substance abuse treatment of adolescents (Larson et al. 1997). Residential drug rehabilitation programs, which were dominated by milieu cure models before managed care, have largely been replaced by 12-Step programs and relapse prevention efforts that have restructured drug rehabilitation around specific recovery tasks and the behavioral analysis of drug use. The once-universal 28-day rehabilitation stay is virtually extinct, replaced by a treatment period tailored to the patient's needs.

Drug rehabilitation programs that collaborate with managed care plans have learned to transition their patients to 12-Step programs and community programs that help patients maintain sobriety. This has been a difficult adjustment for programs that retain patients long stable in sobriety, providing a broad psychotherapy in the name of relapse prevention. Some patients may not need this extended rehabilitation treatment; others who could benefit from exploratory psychotherapy cannot receive it effectively within the confines of the concrete treatment that drug rehabilitation programs provide. Under the new paradigm, a rehabilitation program initially succeeds in helping the patient become sober and stay sober, then refers the patient elsewhere for whatever more general psychotherapeutic services are necessary.

Dual Diagnosis Creep

Major depression, anxiety disorders, and many other psychiatric illnesses occur more frequently in patients who abuse substances. Recognizing and treating these disorders may be essential to the patient's sobriety; however, anxiety and depressive symptoms that are secondary to substance abuse often remit during the first weeks of sobriety (Brown et al. 1995; Davidson 1995). Treatment guidelines generally urge clinicians to curb their enthusiasm for identifying and treating concurrent psychiatric illnesses: "The acute and chronic pharmacological effects of abused substances can mimic most psychiatric symptoms. It is important, therefore, that the clinician observe the patient during a period of abstinence, or have a valid report of symptoms during a period of abstinence, before making a diagnosis of comorbidity" (Buckstein 1997, p. 144S).

While it may be tempting to label patients as "dual diagnosis" or "MICA" (mentally ill chemically dependent) in order to secure approval for higher levels of care, this "diagnosis creep" can mislead patients into attributing their difficulties to other psychiatric illnesses rather than to substance abuse disorders. Primary substance abusers in recovery embrace the straightforward mandate to bear one's affects without recourse to exogenous chemicals; however, recovering MICA patients treated with psychopharmacotherapeutic drugs must learn to distinguish their "bearable" affects from others that warrant pharmacotherapeutic management. MICA patients must also battle the seductive fallacy that pharmacological treatment of their underlying diagnoses will relieve their substance abuse without a struggle to maintain sobriety. The promotion of medical models and pharmacological cures for substance can foster addiction to prescription medications, transform alcoholic individuals into alcoholic sedative abusers, and mislead therapists and patients into denying the need for abstinence from abusable substances.

Adolescence is the time when many chemically dependent patients begin their drug abuse careers. Confronted with adolescent patients exhibiting both mental health and substance abuse problems, therapists must mobilize all their diagnostic acumen to assess if the substance abuse is sufficiently larval to be treatable in psychotherapy, or if it has metamorphosed into the malignant form that requires formal drug rehabilitation treatment. Although this determination can be difficult or impossible, many managed care companies now authorize patients to receive either psychotherapy or drug/alcohol rehabilitation, but not both. Patients who abuse substances may be authorized to receive only two or three individual psychotherapy or family therapy sessions, with these focused on the need to begin attending drug rehabilitation treatment.

To prevent this curtailment of psychotherapy, a clinician may be tempted to minimize the importance of an adolescent's periodic intoxications, misidentifying these as efforts to self-medicate another psychiatric disorder that might remit with psychotherapy, thus eliminating the patient's need to rely on substance abuse. Substance abuse may begin as self-medication, but as it evolves it becomes autonomous, persisting even when the underlying mental diagnosis remits. Therapists who treat adolescents can be seduced by the hope that the substance abuse was "nipped in the bud" and that the teenager need not commit to sobriety or attend drug rehabilitation. These pitfalls are marked by danger signs like the therapist excusing the patient's continued substance use as "only on weekends," "age appropriate," or "not interfering with school work."

For adolescents who can not remain sober, with their sobriety confirmed by family members and by "clean," witnessed, urine toxicology screens, psychotherapy—with or without concurrent psychopharmcotherapy—does not suffice. These adolescents require a dedicated drug/alcohol rehabilitation treatment before, or concurrent with, their psychotherapy/pharmcotherapy treatment. It is a catch-22: patients who can stop using intoxicants may not have to, but those who cannot stop definitely must if psychotherapy is to succeed. If the patient with a mental health problem cannot stop using intoxicants, the substance abuse is a part of his or her mental health problem—or may be provoking most of his or her mental health problem—and must be treated explicitly.

Medication Versus Talking Cures

Pharmacotherapy provides clearer standards for therapeutic dose, frequency, and purity than does psychotherapy, yet the difficulty of providing effective psychotherapy does not warrant the tilt toward pharmacotherapy that pervades the clinical criteria and review practices of many managed care companies. This preference can be explicit in rules specifying that, for example, major depressive disorder can be treated with medication alone but not with psychotherapy alone; or it can be embedded in the practice of peremptorily approving drug treatments while closely scrutinizing psychotherapies.

This bias is especially irrational in treating patients with conditions for which psychotherapy and pharmacotherapy are similarly effective (e.g., in treating patients who have forms of obsessive-compulsive disorder [OCD] that are responsive to behavior therapy) (Frances et al. 1997; Greist 1996). Evidence-based treatment protocols for such patients would favor behavior therapy alone or in combination with pharmacotherapy: patients treated with only pharmacotherapy relapse more frequently once treatment ceases, whereas the improvement persists in many patients who receive behavior therapy and learn to resume their behavior therapy practices, without a therapist, at the first sign of relapse (March and Leonard 1996).

The therapist who is seeking approval for a course of such behavior therapy has to understand how to use the managed care company's procedures. Most managed care companies will approve a few sessions for an initial evaluation and treatment. The behavior therapist who is treating the patient with OCD should use these sessions to demonstrate the efficacy of this treatment, citing the patient's objective signs of improvement to support the request for continuing the behavioral treatment. If that request is denied, the therapist is responsible to appeal the denial (see Chapter 8, this volume). In such cases, the therapist should ask that the appeal be heard by a psychiatrist who is certified in adolescent or child/adolescent psychiatry.

Geographic Cures

Another revolutionary managed care practice is the ban on "geographic treatment"—the treatment of patients at facilities remote from their homes. Why send your child far away for treatment? Parents may prefer an acclaimed treatment facility, or hope to distance the adolescent from "bad company," or may distance themselves from the treatment with an attitude of "send him back when he's fixed." Whatever the motivation, family evaluation and family therapy are usually essential in treating adolescents, and managed care companies routinely insist that adolescents be treated close to home, with parents and other family members attending regularly scheduled sessions for evaluation and family therapy (Bukstein 1997). Yet it is a mistake to exclude all geographic treatments; sometimes a patient already located in a remote location is best treated there in situ.

Case Example

A 17-year-old was sent by his family to live in Israel, hoping this would cure his drug dependence, but it persisted. In Israel he was admitted to a drug rehabilitation program that incorporated a strong religious focus as a spiritual component. It was medically necessary for him to be treated in a residential drug rehabilitation program, the nearest in-network facility was 6,000 miles away, and the cost of his treatment per day was inexpensive by United States standards, so his stay was approved, his care was managed, and he did well.

Managed care companies should respond more flexibly when students develop an episode of mental illness while attending college far from home. Colleges are reexamining their tradition of automatically sending home students who develop significant psychiatric symptoms while in school. Although the school eliminates its own risk by sending the student home, it is wiser to assess this on a case-by-case basis, since the student sent home may become embroiled in exactly the same family cauldron that generated his or her pathology and impedes recovery. The managed care company must be prepared to treat college students where they attend school. In college communities, it is best to use practitioners familiar with mobilizing support systems in the academic setting: sometimes, for example, patients can be sent out on passes to attend class while temporarily residing in the college infirmary (Lipschitz 1990).

Medical Necessity

Managed care companies uniformly authorize only treatments that are "medically necessary," but this term has radically different meanings to doctors and to insurers (Rosenbaum et al. 1999). Within the insurance industry, commercial insurers, Medicare, and the various Medicaid programs use different definitions of "medical necessity," and its meaning varies from state to state, depending on court rulings, state regulations, and local administrative decisions (Bergthold 1995; Simon 1997). Most commercial insurers use a similar definition, specifying that a treatment is medically necessary when:

1. The patient has a psychiatric illness that a) is described in DSM-IV (American Psychiatric Association 1994) and b) is severe enough to impair the patient's functioning; and
2. The treatment provided a) is the treatment most likely to be effective for this condition, b) has the goal of improving the condition or preventing its worsening, and c) is provided in the least restrictive environment, so that the level of care corresponds to the severity of the behavioral impairment.

Treatments are commonly rejected when the managed care company judges that the patient's illness is not severe enough or that the treatment does not meet these criteria. Many companies, for example, will approve pharmacotherapy for generalized anxiety disorder or major depression but deny approval for psychotherapy for these conditions, asserting that pharmacotherapy is the treatment more likely to be effective.

Like most managed care standards and practices, this model of medical necessity initially evolved in managing the treatments provided to employees of large corporations. Managed care companies channeled these patients into treatments that ameliorated their acute crises and restored them to their previous level of function. These treatments focused on patients' objective signs of impairment and sidestepped their underlying character styles and chronic behavior patterns. This approach implicitly posited the patient's characteristic long-term behavior as their healthy, desirable, "normal" state.

This focus on the symptoms currently pressing in the here and now helped the patient and the therapist avoid digressing into areas the insurer considered less relevant to the immediate medical needs of the patient. Pursuing this pragmatic agenda also reassured prospective patients who feared that psychiatric treatment could compel a global reexamination and reevaluation of their lives.

Although this narrow treatment focus often succeeded with the corporate employees who were the prototypical managed care patients, managed care organizations have gradually recognized that patients who have more severe, chronic, and persistent impairment may require broadening the scope of treatment efforts. Suicidal thoughts, threats, or acts are often recurring symptoms of a chronic and persistent illness that is marked by remissions and exacerbations. Patients who were once suicidal may continue to need treatment after remission of their acute objective signs of suicide risk. However, the therapist cannot hope to demonstrate that the patient's current treatment is effective simply by citing symptoms the patient once presented or stressors from the patient's history. The therapist must show that the patient both has improved with treatment and is continuing to improve with treatment. Therapists treating these patients must learn how to recognize and report the signs that demonstrate that the patient is making progress in the course of the therapy.

Excluded Conditions and Treatments

Managed care organizations typically exclude from coverage all treatments that are not necessary for the psychiatric care of the patient, even though these treatments may be mandated by courts, parole officers, schools, wives, husbands, parents, employers, or employee assistance programs. Educational testing and remedial education are not covered by the patient's medical insurance, and the costs for these services are shifted to patients' school districts.

The list of exclusions varies from company to company, but mental health insurance coverage typically excludes marital therapy, sex therapy, smoking cessation treatment, treatment of injuries resulting from military combat (i.e., posttraumatic stress disorders due to military trauma), and a smorgasbord of other conditions and treatments. The exclusions are listed both in the provider manual distributed to participating treatment "providers" by the managed care organizations and in the plan benefit summary that the insurance company gives to subscribers. Therapists starting treatment with any new patient should consult their provider manual or the patient's plan benefit summary in order to help plan the treatment. Therapists should discuss with patients and their families any treatment restrictions resulting from insurance limitations. Of course, it is important to present these restrictions in ways that do not undermine the patient's confidence in the treatment he or she receives from his or her provider.

Medical or Psychiatric?

Companies commonly exclude "medical" conditions from coverage in the mental health benefit. Such "medical" exclusions can include attention-deficit/hyperactivity disorder; pervasive developmental disorders, including autistic disorder and its subtypes; and Tourette's syndrome. Although treatment of these conditions is excluded, most companies will cover acute psychiatric complications superimposed on these underlying illnesses. Case managers are frequently unaware of this, and it is often useful to appeal their denials of medical treatments.

Case Example

A 16-year-old girl who had never received psychiatric treatment was admitted for an episode of acute mania that was attributed to corticosteroids administered to treat a flare-up of her systemic lupus erythematosus. The case manager denied coverage for the stay, but the facility appealed this determination, noting that she was receiving a psychiatric treatment provided by a psychiatrist in a psychiatric inpatient unit. The managed care company's consultant psychiatrist reversed the denial and approved the treatment, noting that the behavioral health insurance would not cover treatment of the underlying medical condition, but would cover treatment of this acute psychiatric complication.

Behavioral managed care companies will more often accept responsibility for approving treatment of a medically ill patient when the patient is given a psychiatric diagnosis and treated by a psychiatrist in a psychiatric hospital. If the managed care company continues to assert that the disease being treated is "medical and not psychiatric," the therapist should present the claim to the carrier of the patient's medical insurance. If the medical carrier denies the claim, that denial should be appealed through its appeal system. In equivocal cases, the medical directors of the plans providing behavioral and medical insurance will have to confer to decide which plan is responsible for covering the treatment. This conference is more likely to occur if the therapist persists in appealing the case.

Family Treatment

Treating families under managed care poses special problems. It is usually essential for therapists who are treating children or adolescents also to evaluate the patients' parents, and their continued couples therapy is sometimes necessary (King 1995); however, many managed care plans entirely exclude marital therapy from coverage. In presenting the case to the managed care company, the therapist has to keep clear which family member is the focus of the therapy. The therapist must carefully show that the couples sessions are not marital therapy "for the couple," but are actually dedicated to resolving issues that concern the child who is the designated patient. Of course, sometimes treating the child requires treating a parent who is depressed, is abusing substances, or has other problems. There is a hazard here if the therapist undertakes to treat different members of the same family, designating each as a primary patient: treating multiple members of the same family often triggers alarms in the managed care company, leading to detailed review of the therapist's practice pattern.

Insurers can produce a different problem when treatments they provide to any dependent of a policyholder ("the subscriber") trigger a letter to the "subscriber" reporting the diagnosis, the treatment modality, the name of the facility or therapist, and the number of days or sessions approved. This information can enter divorce proceedings and custody hearings. When the subscriber should not be apprised of this confidential information, the therapist should send the managed care company a written notice describing the problem. The notice should inform them that the consent signed by the separated spouse authorizes disclosures to the insurer but explicitly prohibits redisclosure to the policyholder or to other third parties, and that disclosure of information to the policyholder would interfere with treatment, harming the patient and preventing the patient from receiving necessary care.

The Chain of Appeals

Even when a managed care company withholds approval of a treatment—because it is not medically necessary, the patient's condition is "medical" rather than psychiatric, or the disease or treatment is "excluded" from coverage—the therapist is not absolved of the duty to provide proper treatment (see Chapter 8, this volume). Courts in the United States continue to hold the clinician—not the insurer—responsible for providing proper treatment (Geraty et al. 1992).

When a necessary treatment is denied by the managed care company, the therapist is responsible for understanding the basis of the denial and appealing it (see Chapter 8). If the company denies approval of the therapist's treatment plan, the therapist should appeal the decision and notify the company if evaluation of the treatment plan requires subspecialty expertise that most psychiatrists do not possess. Managed care companies are required to provide these appeals quickly, within days. Companies must provide for at least two levels of appeal after the initial denial. These appeals often succeed, especially when the initial denial came from a case manager who was new or not familiar with treatment standards. The appeal advocates for the patient in a number of ways, not least because of court rulings that patients can obtain judicial review of these decisions—and damages—only after they exhaust the appeals procedure offered by the insurance plan.

Children and adolescents can be alluring patients, and their parents' insurer or employer may be willing to approve treatments that are excluded or denied by their contracted managed care organization. While patients are reluctant to expose their own mental health or substance abuse problem in an appeal to their employer, most parents feel less stigma about exposing their childrens' difficulties in order to have their treatments covered. Parents often have been able to enlist their firm's employee benefits office to advocate on their behalf.

Other clinical circumstances, as well, may warrant involving the employee benefits office. Fostering a positive bond between patient and therapist is an important element in psychotherapy, and this bond may be sundered when a new managed care plan forces a patient to select a new therapist from the limited "panel" of providers whom the plan recruits. Some unfortunate patients have been forced to switch therapists as many times as their employer switched managed care plans. Patients who are battered by such a succession of therapist switches should ask their employee benefits office to instruct the managed care company to enroll their current therapist in the managed care network so that the treatment can continue without setback.

Appeal to the employee benefits office is also warranted when the benefit has been exhausted while the treatment remains effective and medically necessary. This request for providing "extracontractual benefits" is particularly compelling when the therapist can show that giving this benefit *reduces* the cost to the insurer or the employer: for example, when approving continued outpatient treatment in a day hospital program prevents a relapse requiring a costly inpatient stay, or when the cost of mental health treatment demonstrably prevents greater medical care expenses.

Case Example

A 15-year-old boy who was dependent on insulin for control of unstable juvenile-onset (type 1) diabetes exhausted his annual mental health benefit of 30 outpatient treatment sessions. Without additional sessions, he was likely to require more frequent medical readmission for diabetic ketoacidosis. His medical insurer had contracted with an independent "carve out" managed care company to manage behavioral health treatments, and this company was not authorized to extend benefits beyond the 30 sessions. When the patient exhausted his outpatient benefit, the managed care company contacted the medical insurer, who approved additional outpatient sessions, exchanging these for the patient's unused psychiatric inpatient benefit days.

The New Responsibilities

The past 40 years have brought unprecedented advances in the scientific understanding of suicide and its risk factors. Yet these same 40 years have witnessed a marked increase in adolescent suicide, an increase that still continues unabated among black male teenagers. Managed care has now entered this deteriorating situation, radically transforming the treatment of those patients who carry the highest suicide risks.

Managed care accepted two sometimes conflicting missions: to control costs and to improve the outcome of treatment. Behavioral managed care programs have succeeded in cutting the costs of care, but many are only beginning to attempt to improve the quality and outcome of the treatments they manage. These evolving missions have imposed a new structure on patient treatment, a structure that is itself imperfect and evolving. In the early days of managed care, patient treatments "fell between the cracks" as therapists, managed care organizations, and treatment institutions each asserted parochial models of treatment. The ensuing imbroglio clarified each one's responsibility for ensuring that the patient receives necessary care. Therapists learned that they cannot treat patients in vacuo, confident that good and necessary treatments will gain retrospective approval, and then fulminate indignantly when their services go unreimbursed (see the addendum to this chapter for tips on avoiding this outcome). Managed care companies found that they cannot impose novel models of illness and treatment and expect that patients will be either cured or silenced. Treating institutions are learning that they cannot decrease utilization and raise treatment quality simply by mandating staff to work faster. These errors were widespread in the first enthusiasms of the managed care revolution, and patients suffered as a result.

If it is mishandled now, this continuing revolution could further raise the suicide rate—if the exigencies of managed care drive therapists, facilities, and insurers to the wholesale curtailment of necessary admissions and stays, heedless of the consequences. Yet the managed care revolution holds a potential for good that is equally revolutionary: insurers can promulgate evaluation standards and treatment procedures that incorporate emerging scientific advances, and providers can respond by more effectively evaluating patients, formulating behavioral treatments, and speeding transitions to lower levels of care.

This rosy scenario requires that the participants stay focused on improving treatment outcomes while accepting new, broader responsibilities for patient care. For therapists, this means hastening patient evaluations by contacting collaterals; understanding which treatments are covered under patients' benefits; delivering clear, focused presentations of targeted treatments to gain approval by managed care companies; and appealing erroneous denial decisions. For treating institutions, ensuring good outcomes means supervising the pace and quality of patient evaluations and treatments, coordinating staff contacts with managed care companies, and providing ready connections to step-down levels of care. For managed care companies, it means ensuring that a well-trained professional staff utilizes authoritative criteria to closely monitor and actively manage the quality and pace of treatment. Accepting these new tasks and new roles will be essential if we are to improve the care of suicidal adolescents in particular and the quality of behavioral care in general.

References

American Psychiatric Association: Diagnostic and Statistical Manual of Mental Disorders, 4th Edition. Washington, DC, American Psychiatric Association, 1994

Bell CC, Clark DC: Adolescent suicide. Pediatr Clin North Am 45:365–380, 1998

Bergthold LA: Medical necessity: do we need it? Health Aff (Millwood) 14:180–190, 1995

Brent DA, Perper JA, Allman CJ: Alcohol, firearms, and suicide among youth: temporal trends in Allegheny County, Pennsylvania, 1960 to 1983. JAMA 257:3369–3372, 1987

Brent DA, Perper JA, Moritz G, et al: Psychiatric risk factors for adolescent suicide: a case-control study. J Am Acad Child Adolesc Psychiatry 3:521–529, 1993

Brown SA, Inaba RK, Gillin JC, et al: Alcoholism and affective disorder: clinical course and depressive symptoms. Am J Psychiatry 152:45–52, 1995

Bukstein O: American Academy of Child and Adolescent Psychiatry. Practice parameters for the assessment and treatment of children and adolescents with substance use disorders. J Am Acad Child Adolesc Psychiatry 36(no. 10, suppl):140S–156S, 1997

Centers for Disease Control: Attempted suicide among high school students—United States, 1990. MMWR Morb Mortal Wkly Rep 40:633, 1991

Centers for Disease Control: Suicide contagion and the reporting of suicide: recommendations from a national workshop. MMWR Morb Mortal Wkly Rep 43(RR-6):9–18, 1994

Centers for Disease Control: Youth risk behavior surveillance—United States, 1995. MMWR Morb Mortal Wkly Rep 45(SS-4):41, 1996

Centers for Disease Control: Suicide among black youths—United States, 1980–1995. MMWR Morb Mortal Wkly Rep 47:193–196, 1998

Clark DC: Suicidal behavior in childhood and adolescence: recent studies and clinical implications. Psychiatric Annals 23:271–275, 1993

Davidson KM: Diagnosis of depression in alcohol dependence: changes in prevalence with drinking status. Br J Psychiatry 166:199–204, 1995

Fowler RC, Rich CL, Young D: San Diego Suicide Study, II: substance abuse in young cases. Arch Gen Psychiatry 43:962–965, 1986

Frances A, Docherty JP, Kahn DA: Treatment of obsessive-compulsive disorder. The Expert Consensus Panel for Obsessive-Compulsive Disorder. J Clin Psychiatry 58 (suppl 4):2–72, 1997

Geraty RD, Hendren RL, Flaa CJ: Ethical perspectives on managed care as it relates to child and adolescent psychiatry. J Am Acad Child Adolesc Psychiatry 31:398–402, 1992

Gould M, Fisher P, Parides M, et al: Psychosocial risk factors of child and adolescent completed suicide. Arch Gen Psychiatry 53:1155–1164, 1996

Greenhill LL, Waslick B: Management of suicidal behavior in children and adolescents. Psychiatr Clin North Am 20:641–666, 1997

Greist JH: New developments in behaviour therapy for obsessive-compulsive disorder. Int Clin Psychopharmacol 11 (suppl 5):63–73, 1996

Guyer B, Lescohier I, Gallagher SS, et al: Intentional injuries among children and adolescents in Massachusetts. N Engl J Med 321:1584–1589, 1989

Hendin H: Psychodynamics of suicide, with particular reference to the young. Am J Psychiatry 148:1150–1158, 1991

Hendin H: Suicide in America, New and Expanded Edition. New York, WW Norton, 1995

King CA, Segal H, Kaminski K, et al: A prospective study of adolescent suicidal behavior following hospitalization. Suicide Life Threat Behav 25:327–338, 1995

King RA. American Academy of Child and Adolescent Psychiatry: Practice parameters for the psychiatric assessment of children and adolescents. J Am Acad Child Adolesc Psychiatry 34:1386–1402, 1995

Larson MJ, Samet JH, McCarty D: Managed care of substance abuse disorders: implications for generalist physicians. Med Clin North Am 81:1053–1069, 1997

Lipschitz A: College Suicide—A Review Monograph. New York, American Suicide Foundation, 1990

March JS, Leonard HL: Obsessive-compulsive disorder in children and adolescents: a review of the past 10 years. J Am Acad Child Adolesc Psychiatry 35:1265–1273, 1996

National Center for Health Statistics: Advance report of final mortality statistics, 1994. Monthly Vital Statistics Report 45 (suppl 3), 1996

Pfeffer CR, Plutchik R, Mizruchi MS, et al: Suicidal behavior in child psychiatric inpatients and outpatients and in nonpatients. Am J Psychiatry 43:733–738, 1986

Restifo K, Shaffer D: Identifying the suicidal adolescent in Primary Care settings. Primary Psychiatry 4:26–34, 1997

Rich CL, Sherman M, Fowler RC: San Diego Suicide Study: the adolescents. Adolescence 25:855–865, 1990

Rosenbaum S, Frankford DM, Moore B, et al: Who should determine when health care is medically necessary? N Engl J Med 340:229–232, 1999.

Shaffer D, Garland A, Gould M, et al: Preventing teenage suicide: a critical review. J Am Acad Child Adolesc Psychiatry 27:675–687, 1988

Shaffer D, Gould M, Fisher P, et al: Psychiatric diagnoses in child and adolescent suicide. Arch Gen Psychiatry 53:339–349, 1996b

Simon RI: Discharging sicker, potentially violent psychiatric inpatients in the managed care era: standard of care and risk management. Psychiatric Annals 27:726–733, 1997

Addendum: Ten Tips for Treating Suicidal Adolescents in Managed Care

1. **Perform a rapid initial evaluation to construct a provisional treatment plan.** Few managed care plans approve extensive evaluation of the patient before beginning treatment; most authorize only one or two evaluation sessions. These insurers may approve further sessions after they receive a report that describes the patient's symptoms and diagnosis and outlines the expected treatment plan. As a first report, it is understood that the plan it describes is provisional and temporary and that it will evolve as the therapist uncovers new information. This initial report should include any important uncertainties and conditions to rule out, and it should specify the information that will be obtained in order to resolve the diagnostic and therapeutic uncertainties.

2. **Promptly gather data from the patient's family members and previous therapists.** Managed care's emphasis on rapid assessment and prompt treatment planning makes it essential that contact with the patient's collaterals and previous therapists occur early in the treatment. Be sure to check the diagnoses that were given to the patient, the patient's adherence to treatment recommendations, and the patient's response to specific medications and to other treatments.
3. **Evaluate suicide risk factors.** Use the information provided by the patient, his or her family members, and other therapists to assemble a careful history of the patient's suicidal thoughts and acts (see Appendix A, this volume, for a further discussion of evaluating suicide risk). Be sure to address the following questions:

    - Which stressors have provoked suicidal thoughts, impulses, and behaviors?
    - What methods did the patient use in suicide attempts, and how lethal were these?
    - How readily were the patient's suicide attempts discovered by others?
    - What premonitory signs heralded these suicide attempts, and how did the patient and his collaterals respond to these warnings?
    - Has another person's suicide provided a model for imitation?
    - What has been the patient's attitude toward suicide? Is it seen as a means of revenge? reunion? rebirth?
    - What dangerous elements are present in the patient's current situation? Is the patient facing some painful humiliation or loss?
    - Does the patient have access to guns, pills, or other lethal temptations?

4. **Focus the treatment report to speak the language of managed care.** Managed care companies review the patient assessment and treatment plan in order to determine if the patient's condition requires treatment, if the patient is receiving the correct treatment, and if the patient could be treated with a less frequent ("less intensive") treatment. This review requires a very specific report that carefully addresses these issues, like the closely focused reports that are used to decide if patients are disabled or competent to prepare a will or stand trial. It is neither necessary nor useful to present a broad biopsychosocial analysis of the patient. Be sure your report targets the patient's dangerous behaviors and thoughts, objective signs of illness, and impairments in the patient's function.

5. **Why now?** It is a managed care credo that treatment must focus on the "Why now?" Did some acute event precipitate the patient's worsening? Look carefully in the patient's history to find some recent development that preceded the exacerbation of the patient's symptoms. In presenting the case to the managed care company, distinguish between the patient's chronic, interepisode behaviors and his or her acute deterioration. Be careful to show that the treatment primarily addresses the patient's acute deterioration while strengthening the patient's defenses and altering his or her environment to limit recurrences.
6. **Determine the potential seriousness of the patient's symptoms.** What is the worst possible outcome to anticipate and avoid? When the patient has been stressed in the past, how severe were the behavioral symptoms that developed? Did he or she become suicidal? psychotic? unable to function at school? The potential seriousness of the patient's symptoms is one factor that enters into the insurer's determination of whether treatment is "medically necessary" to forestall or prevent relapse.
7. **Show that continuing treatment is necessary, that it has been effective, and that it continues to be effective.** Historical data are not sufficient to establish that the patient currently requires the proposed treatment: that the patient once sustained some trauma or in the past had some symptoms suggests that the patient may be at risk of developing symptoms, but this historical information does not show that treatment is necessary now. Patients' symptoms may initially respond to treatment or partially remit but then plateau and not improve further as the treatment continues. The treatment continues to be necessary when the patient continues to have symptoms that require treatment and when these symptoms improve as treatment continues. To show that the current treatment is necessary, describe how the former symptoms improved with treatment and how the remaining symptoms now continue to improve.

    If the patient is receiving a maintenance treatment that is not expected to further reduce his or her symptoms but is necessary to prevent relapse, it is necessary to show that this treatment is provided at the lowest intensity of care that suffices to prevent the patient's worsening. To demonstrate this most effectively, show that efforts to provide less intensive treatment have led to the patient's worsening and loss of his or her gains.
8. **Plan early to step down the intensity of the treatment.** The first phase of treatment may require much effort to organize a clear picture of the

patient's symptoms, gather history, establish diagnosis, present a treatment plan to the patient and family, and determine whether the treatment is effective. Stabilizing the patient during this initial phase may require an intensive level of outpatient or inpatient treatment. However, once the patient clearly is improving with treatment, the treatment intensity can often be reduced: outpatients may be seen less frequently, and inpatients may be stepped down to lower levels of care. With time, as their improvement slows and their condition plateaus, the treatment goal shifts away from improvement and toward maintenance of the gains that were achieved and relapse prevention. This maintenance phase usually requires a still lower intensity of treatment.

The therapist should anticipate these step-downs and should prepare the patient well in advance. Patients should be transitioned from inpatient units when they are well enough to be treated in day ("partial") hospital programs; they can no longer expect to continue inpatient treatment until they improve enough to be treated with a weekly or biweekly visit to a psychiatrist's office. Outpatients should expect to transition to shorter and less-frequent sessions as they improve. When a patient shows that he or she cannot be safely stepped down to a less intensive treatment, be prepared to justify this to the managed care organization by detailing the signs that are preventing or delaying the step-down and by describing the specific hazard of prematurely reducing the intensity of the patient's treatment.

9. **Know the exclusions and limitations of the patient's insurance plan.** Before submitting the authorization request, look through the manual that the plan gives to mental health treatment providers or the summary of benefits booklet the plan gives to patients. Make sure the treatment meets the managed care organization's definition of "medical necessity." Be certain that you are not requesting treatment for some diagnosis that is excluded from coverage. What are the limits of the coverage? Does the patient have insurance benefits to cover the number of treatment sessions or days that you expect he or she will require? If the patient requires a treatment that is not covered, or will need more sessions than their insurance allows, explain to the patient the limitations of his or her insurance coverage. Plan with the patient what to do about the noncovered sessions—whether the patient will pay you for them, or go elsewhere to receive them at a lower cost, or do without.

10. **Request an appeal when approval for medically necessary treatment is denied.** If the managed care organization denies approval for a treatment you consider medically necessary, request an appeal. An appeal is

not a waste of time: often, authorizations are denied by case managers simply because they are given insufficient information to permit their approving the treatment. Companies are contractually obligated to resolve requests to appeal denials of ongoing treatment rapidly. If the therapist does not appeal the denial, lawsuits and other avenues of redress are usually closed to patients.

CHAPTER 5

Suicide in the Elderly

Ashok Bharucha, M.D.

The emergence of managed health care delivery systems in the United States has posed significant clinical challenges, particularly in the area of mental health. A powerful mandate for effective use of resources has inevitably led to concerns about the rationing and quality of mental health care provided by current insurance plans. The scarcity of systematic outcome studies for most psychiatric interventions, on the other hand, has undermined the ability of policy-makers to design cost-effective, research-based treatment protocols that emphasize the health gains per dollar spent. Indeed, the reconciliation of efficient resource needs with the provision of effective treatment is the daunting task faced by managed care organizations.

Some of the most complex interactions between economic, social, and clinical forces in mental health care must be considered in a discussion of late-life depression and its dire potential outcome of suicide. Many managed care organizations have sought to control costs by assigning the management of patients with major depressive disorders to primary care clinicians or by making them the gatekeepers to mental health specialists. Although this strategy may prove to be advantageous to those individuals who are reluctant to seek help from mental health specialists and addresses the potential problem of overestimation of psychopathology by specialists, current literature on major depression and suicidal behavior calls for caution rather than enthusiasm about this approach and stresses the need for further evaluation of this model of mental health care delivery. For example, the diagnosis of depression is said to be missed in no less than half of depressed patients in the general medical setting (D. Goldberg et al. 1982; Kessler et al. 1985a, 1985b; Nielsen and Williams 1980; Schwab et al. 1967; Seller et al. 1981; Sheperd et al. 1966; Wells 1985). Furthermore, even accurate diagnosis in primary care settings is often followed by inadequate doses and duration of antidepressant treatment (Katon et al. 1992; Wells et al. 1994). Extending the argument, the communication of suicidal thoughts is reported to be significantly less common in the primary care setting than in the psychiatric setting (Isometsa et al. 1994a; Murphy 1975)—a point of great clinical relevance in the management of patients with late-life major depression and suicidal behavior.

The impact of managed health care delivery systems on the management of late-life depression and suicidal behavior is reviewed here in the context of what is known about the epidemiology, biology, and pathology associated with late-life suicide. The detection and management of mood disorders, the most common antecedent to late-life suicide, are addressed as the salient points of intervention. Preventative strategies focusing on psychoeducation, community outreach, and liaison with suicide prevention centers are also discussed as cost-effective, quality-of-life enhancing methods to be systematically studied and, it is to be hoped, supported by managed care organizations.

Epidemiology of Suicide

Suicide ranked as the ninth leading cause of death in the United States in 1992, with 30,484 deaths and a suicide rate of 12.0 per 100,000 population according to the mortality statistics of the National Center for Health Statistics (NCHS) (Kochanek and Hudson 1995). The suicide rate was highest among those over the age of 65 years (19.1 per 100,000) and remarkably high in the 75–84 years age group (22.8 per 100,000) (Kochanek and Hudson 1995). As a context for comparison, the elderly (65+ years) constituted 12.6% of the U.S. population in 1992 and yet accounted for 20.2% of the suicides, whereas those in the 15–24 year age group constituted 14.2% of the population and committed 15.4% of the suicides (McIntosh 1995b).

Demographic analysis of these data reveals four crucial variables correlated with late-life suicide rates: sex, race, marital status, and method of suicide attempt. Of these, disparity along gender lines is the most striking, with U.S. males completing suicide four times as often as females in 1992 (McIntosh 1995b). The addition of Caucasian race as a demographic factor further amplifies the risk to 22,126 deaths by white males in that year (Kochanek and Hudson 1995). Whereas the suicide risk for white males is incremental with advancing age, that for Hispanic, African, and Native Americans is reported to peak by early adulthood and decline thereafter (McIntosh et al. 1994). With the exception of the high-risk group of young widowers, the suicide rate in each marital category is also noted to be higher in the elderly (McIntosh et al. 1994). Finally, the elderly, both male and female, are more likely to use firearms as the method of suicide than younger individuals. In 1992, 68.7% of elderly suicides were completed with firearms, compared with approximately 60% of all U.S. suicides (McIntosh 1995b). Males used firearms seven times more frequently than did females, while females outnumbered males in using solid or liquid poisons (McIntosh 1995b).

Although the overall suicide rate for the U.S. adult population has remained relatively stable since World War II, the trend of late-life suicide is notable for a decline by more than 50% from the Great Depression to the lowest recorded rate of 17.1 in 1981 (McIntosh et al. 1994). McIntosh speculates the diminution to be primarily a result of fewer suicides by males, specifically white males; a larger cohort of women; and period effects such as increased political and social activism, economic security, and medical/psychiatric advancements (McIntosh et al. 1994). In contrast, however, the 1980s witnessed an alarming rise of 20% in the elderly suicide rate (McIntosh et al. 1994). Because older Americans constitute an increasingly larger portion of the total population, this increased suicide rate implies large increases (as much as 40%) in the absolute number of late-life suicides (McIntosh et al. 1994). While improved data collection and reporting has been thought to account for some fraction of the recently reported rise in late-life suicide rates, the political and economic insecurity of the last decade are likely more important factors as was the case during the Great Depression in the 1930s (McIntosh et al. 1994).

The prediction of the future suicide rates presents an enormous challenge given the multiple socioeconomic, political, and historical forces that may impinge on the lives of older Americans (McIntosh et al. 1994). Notwithstanding the period effects, it is well known that the suicide rates in each age group have been higher for the "baby boomers" than did their prior cohorts (Manton et al. 1987; McIntosh et al. 1994; Pollinger-Haas and Hendin 1983); furthermore, official suicide statistics reflect only those deaths that in fact have been confirmed to be self-inflicted. As Osgood and Brant (1990) point out, many elderly refuse food and medications and have "accidents." It is unclear what percentage of deaths attributed to other causes are truly suicides. The problem is confounded further since only 20% of long-term care facilities record and report suicides (Osgood and Brant 1990). However speculative the current data, the implications warrant the attention of health care policy-makers.

By the year 2030, McIntosh predicted that Americans over the age of 65 years will make up 20% of the U.S. population and will account for a staggering one-third of all U.S. suicides if current trends continue (McIntosh et al. 1994). Future research on the epidemiology of late-life suicide should focus on establishing 1) international classification criteria for suicidal behavior and completed suicides, 2) the effect on late-life suicide rates of limiting access to firearms, and 3) improving and standardizing the documentation of suicidal behaviors in long-term care facilities.

Biology of Suicide

The identification of individuals at high risk of suicide is a priority if preventive and treatment measures are to be implemented. The limited value of demographic and clinical parameters in predicting suicidal behavior has propelled the current interest in identifying biological correlates of suicidal behavior (Mann and Arango 1992; Pandey et al. 1995). Although the study of the biology of self-injurious behavior was initially conceptualized through an extension of biological research on depression, Winchel and colleagues (1990) now argue for a reconceptulization of self-injurious behavior as a distinct entity on the following grounds: 1) stability of the suicide rate despite new treatments for specific psychiatric disturbances, 2) occurrence of suicide across a spectrum of psychiatric diagnoses, and 3) biochemical findings correlated with suicidal behavior rather than with specific psychiatric diagnoses.

In 1976 Åsberg and colleagues reported a bimodal distribution of cerebrospinal fluid (CSF) 5-hydroxyindoleacetic acid (5-HIAA) in their group of depressed patients, of whom those with low CSF 5-HIAA concentrations were significantly more prone to attempt suicide and to use more violent means. Since then much of the research on the biological markers of suicidal behavior has focused on dysregulation of the serotonergic system. Well beyond the scope of this chapter, a comprehensive review of the neuroendocrine and neurotransmitter studies of suicidal behavior can be found in a paper by Bharucha and Satlin (1997). In the only study to date to investigate the possibility of biological markers of suicidal behavior in the elderly, Jones and colleagues (1990) reported significantly lower concentrations of CSF 5-HIAA and homovanillic acid (HVA) in suicidal than in nonsuicidal patients and control subjects, while no significant differences were detected on psychosocial, psychological, or behavioral measures.

Future progress in identifying biological markers of late-life suicide has been hampered by the limited and often contradictory data on the effect of aging on central nervous system (CNS) neurotransmitter systems and by the difficulty in classifying many elderly deaths as suicide when passive means are used. In addition, however, a number of complex methodological flaws in biological research on suicide need to be addressed as outlined by van Praag (1986): 1) differentiating self-mutilative from suicidal behaviors, 2) establishing a relationship between the lethality of attempt and the lethality of intent, 3) standardizing the timing of biological tests, 4) analyzing data from past and recent suicide attempters separately, 5) classifying biological test results according to the phenomenology of the suicidal behavior, and 6) specifying the degree of impulsivity versus premeditation just as the distinction violent versus nonviolent act has often been made.

Physical Illness and Suicide

A number of studies have investigated age-related variations in recent life events preceding suicide (Carney et al. 1994; Conwell et al. 1990; Heikkinen et al. 1995; Rich et al. 1991). While family, occupational, and financial problems seem to be a more common stressor in younger suicide victims, somatic illness has been noted to be a more common stressor in elderly suicides, a finding that is in keeping with earlier observations (Chynoweth et al. 1980; Darbonne 1969; Dorpat et al. 1968; Jarvis and Boldt 1980; Kwan 1988; Robins 1981; Robins et al. 1959; Sainsbury 1955, 1962, 1963; Whitlock 1986). More specifically, Rich and colleagues (1991) found medical illness to be the most frequent stressor in suicide victims over the age of 80 years. Although most studies lack age- and sex-specific control groups, there is also a preliminary suggestion of higher rates of physical illness in older men who commit suicide compared with older women who commit suicide (Chia 1979; Chynoweth 1981; Dorpat et al. 1968; Heikkinen et al. 1995; Whitlock 1986). Paralleling the findings in suicide completers, physical illness is also a common stressor in older suicide attempters (Kontaxakis et al. 1988; Lester and Beck 1974; Lyness et al. 1992; Sendbuehler and Goldstein 1977).

The nature of the association between specific physical ailments and increased suicide risk has been confounded by several methodological problems. Stenager and Stenager (1992) have classified these into the following general categories: 1) type of investigation (autopsy vs. follow-up vs. epidemiological), 2) population investigated, 3) suitability of control groups, 4) epidemiological/statistical methods used, and 5) validity of suicide statistics presented. In spite of the methodological limitations of the research, increased suicide risk has been reported in both neurological and non-neurological conditions. Mackenzie and Popkin (1987) reviewed the literature on suicide in the medical patient and reported the following CNS conditions to be associated with an increased suicide risk: multiple sclerosis, epilepsy, Huntington's disease, traumatic spinal lesions, and cranial trauma. The authors reported similar findings for non-CNS conditions such as peptic ulcer disease, rheumatoid arthritis, cardiopulmonary diseases, renal disease requiring chronic hemodialysis, and chronic pain (Mackenzie and Popkin 1987).

The research findings assessing the risk of suicide in patients with malignancies have been inconsistent, with some supporting an association (Campbell 1966; Farberow et al. 1963; Fox et al. 1982; Louhivuori and Hakama 1979; Marshall et al. 1983; Whitlock 1978) and others refuting this claim, particularly in hospitalized cancer patients (Bolund 1985a, 1985b; Filiberti et al. 1991; Hietanen and Lonnqvist 1991). In summarizing the literature on the risk of suicide in patients with cancer, Mackenzie and Popkin (1987) suggested that males with cancer are particularly vulnerable to suicide as long as 5 years after diagnosis. Chemotherapy and nonlocalized disease as well correlate with higher risk (Mackenzie and Popkin 1987).

Psychopathology of Late-Life Suicide

According to 1989 statistics, only 3% of the total Medicare budget was consumed by mental health services, of which less than 0.5% was spent on services for noninstitutionalized elderly persons (Shea 1998; Sherman 1992). Despite this relatively small expenditure for mental health services for the elderly, the rising cost of health care has led even Medicare to provide managed care options, the most common of which is the Medicare risk contract (MRC), in which capitated payments are made to health plans for their enrollees (Eisdorfer 1995). Indications are that as many as 80,000 Medicare beneficiaries per month are subscribing to MRCs, with an expected growth by year 2005 of 22%–29% of all eligible Medicare recipients (Colenda and Sherman 1998; Eisdorfer 1995).

The impact of such a system of health care financing on the ability of the elderly to access mental health services remains to be seen. Indeed, the true health and fiscal advantages of managed care plans will only be realized to the extent that they effectively remove barriers to care such as limited referrals to specialists, lengthy and cumbersome preauthorization procedures for services, inattention to the transportation needs of the elderly, and the potential fragmentation of medical and psychiatric care in managed care "carve-out" systems (Colenda et al. 1998; Physician Payment Review Commission 1997).

Historically, there has been an unfortunate separation in the provision of general medical and mental health services in the United States. R. J. Goldberg (1996) posits the following factors to be critical in leading to this separation: a system of specialists fragmenting the care, persisting mind-body dualism, differences in language and practice styles between mental health and medical care providers, common geographic separation of mental health programs from medical settings, stigma of mental illness, medical providers' general discomfort with mental health issues because of insufficient psychiatric training, and carve-out models of psychiatric care that further bifurcate mental health services from medical care. The immense importance of this artificial separation in the care of the elderly cannot be overstated in light of the fact that the vast majority of the mentally ill elderly receive care from their primary care provider and typically present with somatic concerns (German et al. 1985).

Indeed, the phenomenology and etiology of somatic concerns in the elderly can often be quite elusive as suggested by several reports of suicide victims whose autopsy revealed significantly less pathology than would have been expected from the extent of the victim's somatic preoccupations (Lyness et al. 1992). Clearly, the individual's perception of his or her physical health may be greatly influenced by the presence of psychopathology (Brown et al. 1986). Several studies have highlighted the fact that the majority of suicide victims with serious physical illness also suffer from psychiatric illness (Chynoweth et al. 1980, Conwell et al. 1991; Dorpat et al. 1968; Robins et al. 1959), particularly mood disorders (Brown et al. 1986). Indeed, Barraclough's (1971) emphasis on the high prevalence of mood disturbances in late-life suicide, including even first episodes of major depression, has gained ample support over the last two decades (Carlson 1984; Clark 1991; Conwell et al. 1991; Dorpat and Ripley 1960; Draper 1994; Nieto et al. 1992). Lyness et al.'s (1992) study of elderly suicide attempters suggests that this finding is not confined only to suicide completers, because a vast majority of the attempters in their study also had a major depressive syndrome.

The ability of managed care organizations to detect and effectively treat major depression, then, is critical in limiting the well-documented functional impairment, morbidity, and mortality associated with the disorder (Ackerman et al. 1988; Broadhead et al. 1990; Depression Guideline Panel 1993a, 1993b; Greenberg et al. 1993; Johnson et al. 1992; Katon and Schulberg 1992; Katon et al. 1986; Rice et al. 1990; Rodin and Voshart 1987; Wells et al. 1989b). Although the growing reliance on primary care physicians to provide mental health care presents an opportunity to reach the 50% of patients with psychiatric problems who receive care only in the general medical sector (Regier et al. 1978; Wells et al. 1986b), primary care physicians are reported to detect depression in no more than half of their affected patients (D. Goldberg et al. 1982; Kessler et al. 1985a, 1985b; Nielsen and Williams 1980; Schwab et al. 1967; Seller et al. 1981; Sheperd et al. 1966; Wells 1985). Compounding this problem is the increasingly recognized functional impairment due to even subthreshold depressive symptoms that often elude the primary care physician's examination (Berkman et al. 1986; Broadhead et al. 1990; Coulehan et al. 1990; Johnson et al. 1992; Skodol et al. 1994). Furthermore, preliminary evidence emphasizes the challenge for primary care physicians not only of detecting major depression but also of providing effective treatment (Eisenberg 1992; Hoeper et al. 1984; Ormel et al. 1991).

Isometsa et al.'s (1994b) recent examination of a sample representing all suicide completers with current DSM-III-R major depression in Finland in a 1-year period stresses precisely this need for improved detection, treatment, and follow-up of clinically depressed patients. The authors reported that a clear majority of these patients were either undertreated or received no specific treatment for depression. Consistent with previous reports (Barraclough et al. 1974; Chynoweth et al. 1980), only one-third received antidepressant therapy, with virtually all of these patients on subtherapeutic doses. More aggressive somatic therapies, such as psychopharmacological augmentation strategies or electroconvulsive therapy (ECT), as well as broadly defined psychotherapy, were quite uncommon. Interestingly, however, the following sex-specific psychopathology and treatment differences emerged: 1) although both males (67%) and females (88%) had psychiatric histories, only 33% of the males were receiving psychiatric treatment at the time of death as opposed to 65% of the females; 2) 44% of the males had psychoactive substance abuse or dependence problems compared with 8% of the females; 3) males less commonly received antidepressants (21%, vs. 54% of the females) or psychotherapy (16%, vs. 42% of the females); and, finally, (4) only 9% of males and 27% of females had communicated suicidal intent to both family members and treatment organizations. Age-specific findings revealed high physical comorbidity and little psychotherapy received by the "older age group" (>51 years).

A subsequent study by Isometsa et al. (1994a), using data from the same

1-year sample, analyzed patient and treatment characteristics in the contexts of psychiatric, medical, or no care. The authors reported the following salient findings: (1) three-fourths of the suicide victims with major depression treated outside the psychiatric domain were men, whereas 65% of women were in psychiatric care at the time of suicide; 2) suicidal intent was communicated by 59% of the patients in the psychiatric setting but only 19% in the medical setting; 3) 60% of suicide completers in psychiatric care received antidepressant therapy compared with 16% in the medical sector; but 4) the vast majority of patients treated with antidepressants in both psychiatric and medical settings received inadequate doses. Although these findings from Finland await replication, they emphasize the need not only for increased detection and adequate treatment of major depression but also for heightened awareness of the sex- and age-specific psychopathology and treatment characteristics in the various treatment settings.

Bartels et al. (1997) recently examined age-related variations in the diagnosis of depression, treatment by specialty provider, and pharmacotherapy in a cross-sectional chart review study of patients from six health maintenance organizations (HMOs) in the United States. Although depression was identified with equal frequency in the younger (18–64 years) and older (65+ years) age groups, the elderly were more likely to be treated with benzodiazepines and less likely to receive selective serotonin reuptake inhibitor (SSRI) antidepressants—a point of great relevance in light of a recent study which suggests that both psychiatrists and nonpsychiatric physicians are more likely to achieve adequate antidepressant treatment with SSRIs (Shasha et al. 1997). Benzodiazepines were the sole treatment for 16.1% of older adults diagnosed with depression in this study (Bartels et al. 1997). While both groups were referred to specialty mental health providers with equal frequency, the elderly received fewer visits (Bartels et al. 1997).

Does the type of health care delivery system or payment plan affect the detection rate of unipolar depression? Wells and colleagues' (1989a) review of data from the Medical Outcomes Study suggests that patients in the general medical sector with prepayment plans are less likely to have their depression detected or otherwise addressed during a particular visit than those receiving fee-for-service care, supporting the similar claim of a previous study (Wells et al. 1986a). In contrast, no such difference was correlated with payment type among patients of mental health specialists. Interestingly, the type of health care delivery system (single-specialty solo or small group practice, large multispecialty group practice or a HMO) was not thought to be influential in the detection of major depression. These findings must clearly be understood within the context of the limitations of the Medical

Outcomes Study outlined by Wells et al. (1989a): 1) observational design, 2) lack of control for clinician characteristics in the different practice organizations, 3) questionable generalizability of the findings from the sample investigated, 4) awareness of all clinician participants that depression was a condition of focus in the study, 5) controversial nature of the validity of diagnoses derived from the Diagnostic Interview Schedule, and 6) deficiencies in the scope of the patient and clinician screeners for the sake of efficient processing. In summarizing their results, the authors astutely questioned whether improved detection of depression necessarily leads to optimal treatment or, one step further removed, improved functional outcome.

From the standpoint of general health, Ware et al. (1996) recently measured differences in 4-year health outcomes for elderly and poor chronically ill patients treated in a managed care system compared with a traditional fee-for-service plan. Twice as many adults 65 years and older (54%) reported their health had declined after 4 years in a managed care system compared with age-matched control subjects in a fee-for-service plan. Furthermore, only 22% of poor patients treated in the managed care plan, compared with 57% of age- and illness-matched patients in the fee-for-service plan, felt they were in better health after 4 years.

Rogers and associates (1993), using data from the Medical Outcomes Study, measured 2-year outcomes for adult outpatients with major depression under prepaid or fee-for-service financing. Defining limitations in role and physical functioning with the Psychological and Physical Sickness Scales, the authors noted new functional impairments, greater nonadherence to antidepressant treatment over time, and greater switching of payment type in patients of psychiatrists who were initially enrolled in prepaid care plans (average age 42 years) compared with those receiving fee-for-service care (average age 41 years) over 2 years. In marked contrast to Wells et al.'s (1989a) earlier findings, the outcome differences by payment type in the psychiatric group were notably absent in depressed patients of other specialty groups. Although patients under the care of psychiatrists were psychologically sicker, the level of initial sickness was not felt to account for the findings, implicating a primary role of the actual care received in the outcome differences. Rogers et al. are continuing to scrutinize treatment differences in the Medical Outcomes Study to shed further light on outcomes for depression by payment types.

Appropriate recognition and management of depressive disorders appears to be a crucial first step in curbing the late-life suicide rates. Although a vast majority of the elderly who commit suicide are reported to be in the midst of a depressive episode, the evaluation of suicide potential is made more difficult in this population by the fact that they are unlikely to have a prior history of mood disorder (Barraclough 1971; Clark 1991; Conwell 1994; Conwell et al. 1991) or suicidal behavior (Carney et al. 1994; Chia 1979; Conwell et al. 1991; Lester and Beck 1974; Lonnqvist and Achte 1985). Given the greater intent to suicide (Conwell et al. 1991), poorer physical health, and increasing social isolation (McIntosh et al. 1994), it is not surprising that the ratio of attempted to completed suicide drops from 200–300:1 in the young (Curran 1987; McIntire and Angle 1981; Parkin and Stengel 1965) to 4:1 in the elderly (Parkin and Stengel 1965; Stenback 1980). More succinctly put, the first suicide attempt in the elderly may be the last. However, some hope for identifying suicide potential is suggested by the fact that as many as 75% of the elderly are said to have seen their primary care physician within 30 days prior to suicide completion (Clark 1991; Conwell et al. 1991).

Prevention

Suicide in the elderly, ultimately, is not usually a response to one major factor; rather, it is the result of a failure of the sum of sustaining biological, somatic, psychological, and sociological elements. The preceding sections have framed the most ominous demographic scenario as that of an elderly widowed white male with a mood disorder, multiple medical problems, and access to firearms. Although these features characterize many older adults who complete suicide, comprehensive preventative strategies for this population must begin with a thorough assessment of the unique aspects of each individual patient. When properly channeled, such attention to detail conveys a degree of concern and empathy to the elderly, who otherwise often feel neglected in a youth-oriented society and may therefore silence the voice of their despair.

It has been widely reported that the elderly rarely use general suicide hotlines or pursue mental health services (Dew et al. 1987; Felton 1982; Gatz and Smyer 1992; German et al. 1985; Lasoski 1986; McIntosh et al. 1981; Osgood 1985; Redick and Taube 1980). To what extent, however, are crisis prevention centers prepared to accurately assess the risk profile and acuity of a situation and link the caller to further care, especially in light of the conflicting reports of the effectiveness of such centers to date (Frankish 1994; Neimeyer and Pfeiffer 1994)? A recent survey of personnel in 321 American Association of Suicidology (AAS)–listed crisis prevention centers in the United States and Canada examined the training, knowledge, and current practices relevant to prevention of suicide among the elderly (Adamek and Kaplan 1996). The authors reported the following findings: 1) 35%–45% of personnel in these centers felt they did not receive training specific to elder or firearm suicide, 2) only 33% of volunteers/staff and 47% of program managers correctly identified older adults as the age group with the highest suicide rate, 3) 54% of volunteers/staff and 63% of program managers recognized guns as the most common method of suicide for older men, but less than 10% of respondents also knew this to be true of older women; and 4) fewer than one-third of respondents stated they would call the police and fewer than one-fifth indicated they would initiate hospitalization in managing a potential firearm suicide. Clearly, this survey suggests that personnel in crisis prevention centers need to be adequately trained in the recognition of age-specific risk profiles of potential suicide victims and the implementation of interventions appropriate to the perceived acuity of the situation. Fostering a joint psychoeducational collaboration between community crisis prevention centers and managed care organizations may in the long term prove to be both clinically sound and cost-effective.

To address the lack of utilization of crisis prevention hotlines and mental health services by older adults, several innovative programs have been implemented. While there is a hope that they will also prove to be cost-effective over time, data regarding this particular aspect are currently lacking (McIntosh 1995a). In St. Louis, Missouri, Life Crisis Services has instituted the Link-Plus component, a program that elicits referrals primarily from medical and mental health personnel targeting the depressed elderly in crisis. These individuals are then referred to the appropriate services with ongoing telephone contact (McIntosh 1995a). In addition to such crisis intervention methods, the Spokane Community Mental Health Center has developed the Gatekeepers Program whereby community members who routinely come in contact with older persons are instructed by local organizations and businesses in the recognition of elderly at risk for self-harm (McIntosh 1995a). Following referral, an in-home evaluation is arranged, leading to appropriate case management. A similar program now also exists in Dayton, Ohio (McIntosh 1995a).

Respecting the salient needs of this population, the San Francisco Suicide Prevention Center has organized the Center for Elderly Suicide Prevention and Grief Related Services, which not only offers 24-hour crisis intervention, the Friendship Line, but also meets the older adults where they are through the Geriatric Outreach Program (McIntosh 1995a). Home visits, ongoing telephone contact, volunteer assistance with moving, and networking within the local agencies are among its primary functions (McIntosh 1995a).

De Leo et al. (1995) modified the crisis intervention model in their study of the Tele-Help/Tele-Check service. Tele-Help is an alarm system to be activated for assistance, while Tele-Check consists of checking in with the clients twice a week to assess their needs and offer emotional support. Only one suicide was found among 12,135 elderly subjects over a 4-year study period. These results are especially noteworthy because the population was predominantly "old-old" (mean age 79 years) and was characterized by demographic suicide risk factors such as low income, isolation, and potential loss of autonomy. Medical, psychiatric, and substance abuse histories were not systematically collected, however. Interestingly, the same authors reported improved mood scores, fewer general practitioner home visits, and fewer hospitalizations among participants of a previous study who used Tele-Check for at least 6 months than were reported by those awaiting the service or who had just been enrolled (De Leo et al. 1992). Although implicit in their discussion, the cost-effectiveness of this program was not documented with any specific data.

The success of crisis prevention models just summarized will depend to a large extent on their ability to search for evidence of major depression and to engage the depressed individuals in treatment. Indeed, there is a growing recognition of the suffering and economic burden imposed by depressive disorders, as indicated by the formulation of "Depression in Primary Care" clinical practice guidelines by the Agency for Health Care Policy and Research (Depression Guideline Panel 1993a, 1993b). A report indicating reduced frequency of elder suicide after systematic postgraduate education of general practitioners on this topic lends some support for managing at least the uncomplicated cases of major depression in the medical sector (Rutz et al. 1989).

The primary care physician is in an opportune position to improve geriatric mental health by attending to general geriatric care (Jorm 1995; Rabins 1992). Optimal management of cardio- and cerebrovascular diseases, chronic cardiopulmonary conditions, decline in special sensory functions, rehabilitation of chronic disabilities, and effective pain management are likely to reduce the demoralization and functional impairment that older adults experience. Furthermore, a Canadian study suggests that of the elderly patients who present to a psychiatric emergency service with a chief complaint of more than a month's duration, the vast majority had previously seen their primary care physician, usually more than once, for the same complaint (Perez and Blouin 1986). Not only do elderly patients have 20% longer emergency room visits, but they also use more hospital-based resources and are more likely to use ambulances to get there (Baum and Rubenstein 1987;

Beland et al. 1990, 1991). Earlier attention and appropriate management of physical and psychiatric symptoms might avert the need for subsequent costly emergency room services.

Primary care and mental health clinicians should become familiar with the demographic factors correlated with increased suicide. Among elderly patients, suicide risk is enhanced by the following factors:

- Age greater than 65 years
- Male
- White
- Presence of physical illness(es) or subjective sense of physical decline
- Current mood disorder
- Family or personal history of mood disorder or suicide attempts
- Psychosocial stressors
- Lack of social supports
- Access to firearms
- Threat of institutionalization

Recent reports have recommended broadening the scope of the screening process for depression or suicide risk in primary care or other settings by using a depression questionnaire such as the Short Beck Depression Inventory (Beck and Beck 1982), Zung Self-Rating Depression Scale (Zung 1965), General Health Questionnaire (Tarnopolsky et al. 1979), Inventory to Diagnose Depression (Zimmerman and Coryell 1987), Medical Outcomes Study Depression Screener (Burnam et al. 1988), PRIME-MD (Williams and Spitzer 1992), Symptom Driven Diagnostic System (Blacklow et al. 1992), or the short version of the Geriatric Depression Scale (Brody et al. 1995; Butler and Lewis 1995; Sheikh and Yesavage 1986). The cross-sectional presence of depressive symptoms should prompt the primary care physician to elicit a longitudinal psychiatric history to inform treatment decisions or, if clinically uncertain, refer the patient to a psychiatrist for further evaluation. Table 5–1 offers some general suggestions for clinicians of any discipline who are advocating for mental health care of the suicidal elderly in a managed care organization. Of primary importance, in this author's view, is the clear documentation of objective indicators of risk and a willingness to appeal when care is denied (see Appendix A, this volume).

TABLE 5–1. Advocating for managed care services for the suicidal older adult: 10 tips for the clinician

1. Collect and organize data from all relevant collateral sources (e.g., family, nursing staff) prior to negotiating appropriate level of care.
2. Offer objective data where possible rather than subjective impressions (e.g., subject eating only 25% of meals).
3. Document noncompliance with treatment(s) and refusal of food and water.
4. Organize and provide a chronology of failed psychotropic medication trials, summarizing doses and durations of treatments.
5. Report presence and feasibility of suicide plan (if communicated); remember to mention the infrequency with which the elderly communicate suicidal ideation.
6. Document access to firearms.
7. Report unstable medical conditions, decline in functioning, or change in behavior, mood, or cognition.
8. Communicate recent or pending psychosocial changes that may precipitate an emotional crisis (e.g., therapist moving).
9. Integrate all three elements of the biopsychosocial model in formulating the case.
10. Firmly insist on timely appeal of treatment denial if the treatment is clinically indicated.

Psychiatric consultation or referral should definitely be initiated when suicidality, homicidality, or psychosis is suspected. In addition, psychiatric consultation should be strongly considered in the following clinical scenarios (Brody et al. 1995; Butler and Lewis 1995):

- Atypical clinical presentation
- Vague symptoms or multiple somatic complaints disproportionate to the actual ascertained physiopathology
- Comorbid psychiatric conditions (particularly personality disorders)
- Polypharmacy
- Complex medical history
- Active substance abuse
- Bipolar disorder

The availability of psychiatric consultants, however, provides only a partial substitute for the development of primary care competence in managing major depression and suicide risk, since a majority of relevant patients seek treatment only in the general medical sector (Regier et al. 1978; Wells et al. 1986b).

Pratt and colleagues (1991) have developed a 3-hour community and professional education program on depression and suicide in later life that is intended for families, older adults, and service providers. The workshop combines an 18-minute slide show entitled *The Final Course*, a story of Mrs. Murphy, aged 72, with lectures and individual and group activities and discussions. Participants are tested on a 12-item true-false knowledge test and a 6-item behavioral intention scale that measures the likelihood of specific actions participants would take in response to a depressed suicidal older person. The authors reported that program participants showed significant gains in knowledge and in their intent to take appropriate action in support of a depressed person compared with a control group. Training primary care physicians, medical and mental health specialists, ancillary support staff, patients, and families with such a workshop may prove to be clinically invaluable, and ultimately cost-effective, for any medical organization. A selection of the available psychoeducational curricula formulated by prominent suicidologists and guidelines for the management of depressive disorders in the primary care setting are listed in the references for the sake of brevity (Brody et al. 1995; Butler and Lewis 1995; Depression Guideline Panel 1993a, 1993b; McIntosh 1987, 1995a; Osgood 1991).

Little is known about the tertiary prevention strategies that may be effective in dealing with the consequences of suicidal behavior, particularly in the elderly (McIntosh 1995a). Identification and management of self-induced illness from failed suicide attempts, and development of strategies for intervening with family members of the suicidal elderly, remain to be systematically studied.

Conclusion

Suicide remains an unacceptably common alternative to suffering in the lives of older Americans. Epidemiological trends forecast a further increase rather than a diminution in the number of suicides in this population in the foreseeable future. The urgent need for biomedical, psychosocial, and health care delivery research addressing the salient features of late-life suicide cannot be overly emphasized. From a biomedical perspective, future research on geriatric suicidal behavior should focus on 1) further delineating the biological correlates of suicidal behavior, with particular emphasis on the platelet serotonin receptor studies; 2) elucidating the neurobiology of the aging process and how it contributes to affective vulnerability; 3) clarifying the complex interactions between the somatic and psychiatric illnesses; 4) identifying personality traits that may confer vulnerability or resistance to suicide in late life; and 5) understanding age-related variations in the prevalence and phenomenology of Axis I psychopathology in suicide victims. Of course, the findings of such research can only be implemented within a health care delivery system capable of actively integrating biomedical and psychosocial interventions.

The formidable clinical challenges posed by late-life depression and suicide are experienced all the more acutely in an economic environment that focuses on cost containment without sacrificing the quality of care. The diverse array of managed care organizations that have emerged have at their core the following premises: 1) focus on preventative care, 2) initial detection and management of major depression by primary care clinicians, 3) integration of services via computerized records, 4) access as determined by medical necessity to multiple disciplines, 5) active use of community resources, 6) development of screening and treatment protocols, 7) medication accessibility and affordability, and 8) conduction of outcome studies to inform future care.

Given managed care organizations' emphasis on the local population's health and preventative care, strategies targeting early case identification and reduction of morbidity and mortality are of particular interest. In regard to late-life suicide, managed care organizations can play a pivotal role in implementing the following primary prevention efforts: 1) early detection of depression and provision of appropriate treatment; 2) early recognition and treatment of medical problems; 3) education of the general public and health care community about geriatric depression and suicide; 4) attention to the financial, housing, and other psychosocial needs of the elderly population by conducting in-home assessments, geriatric outreach (e.g., daily medication schedule calls), and advocacy with social services, families, and other physicians; 5) support of access (and possibly provision of transportation) to socialization programs such as senior day centers; 6) communication with staff at long-term care facilities to identify and remedy problems early; and 7) advocacy of firearms control.

Secondary prevention strategies should focus on 1) educating the staff of suicide prevention centers in appropriate recognition and triage of at-risk elderly, 2) improving case-finding through use of structured interviews or self-rating scales of depression such as those previously mentioned, 3) using active outreach services such as calls to remind clients of daily medication schedules and networking with social services, 4) involving families in treatment planning, and 5) educating the primary care physicians about the differential diagnosis of mood disorders, pharmacotherapeutic approaches, psychosocial interventions, and appropriate referral decisions and use of specialists. The development of treatment and referral protocols may also assist in designing outcome studies that are crucial to the long-term adoption of an effective program.

Tertiary prevention strategies for dealing with the consequences of suicidal and parasuicidal behavior have been poorly studied, particularly as they relate to the geriatric population, and this has limited the ability to offer cogent management guidelines. Clearly, self-induced illness from failed suicide attempts should be promptly assessed and treated. Family and community resources should be immediately mobilized to address the issues that may have contributed to an individual's decision to attempt suicide. In this regard, a referral to a psychiatrist with regularly scheduled phone sessions in between actual visits seems prudent until the acuity of the situation is deemed to be low by the treatment team. More importantly, primary care physicians need to contact and involve the families of suicide attempters/completers to assess their emotional and medical needs, especially if they were not involved in the patient's treatment planning in the first place.

There are important caveats regarding managed care of the depressed and/or suicidal elderly. The potential advantages of managed care organizations in limiting the morbidity and mortality of parasuicidal/suicidal behaviors in a cost-efficient manner are threatened by pressure to care for patients with shorter visits, long intervisit intervals, reduced referrals to specialists, emphasis on focal complaints, shifting service delivery to less well-trained (and thus less costly) professionals, and potential preference for pharmacotherapy versus psychotherapy. Indeed, feedback mechanisms both from within and from without the managed care organizations are necessary to encourage the highest quality of care as these managed health care delivery systems continue to evolve, spread, and provide care for an increasing proportion of the elderly.

References

Ackerman AD, Lyons JS, Hammer JS, et al: The impact of coexisting depression and timing of psychiatric consultation on medical patients' length of stay. Hospital and Community Psychiatry 39:173–176, 1988

Adamek ME, Kaplan MS: Managing elder suicide: a profile of American and Canadian crisis prevention centers. Suicide Life Threat Behav 26:122–131, 1996

Åsberg M, Thorén P, Träskman L: "Serotonin depression"—a biochemical subgroup within the affective disorders? Science 191:478–480, 1976

Barraclough BM: Suicide in the elderly. Br J Psychiatry 6(suppl):87–97, 1971

Barraclough BM, Bunch J, Nelson B, et al: A hundred cases of suicide: clinical aspects. Br J Psychiatry 125:355–373, 1974

Bartels SJ, Horn S, Sharkey P, et al: Treatment of depression in older primary care patients in health maintenance organizations. Int J Psychiatry Med 27:215–231, 1997

Baum SA, Rubenstein LZ: Old people in the emergency room: age-related differences in emergency department use and care. J Am Geriatr Soc 35:398–404, 1987

Beck AT, Beck RW: Screening depressed patients in family practice: a rapid technique. Postgrad Med 52:81–85, 1982

Beland F, Philibert L, Thouez JP, et al: Socio-spatial perspectives on the utilization of emergency hospital services in two urban territories in Quebec. Soc Sci Med 30:53–66, 1990

Beland F, LeMay A, Philibert L, et al: Elderly patients' use of hospital-based emergency services. Med Care 29:408–418, 1991

Berkman LF, Berkman CS, Kasl S, et al: Depressive symptoms in relation to physical health and functioning in the elderly. Am J Epidemiol 124:372–388, 1986

Bharucha AJ, Satlin A: Late-life suicide: a review. Harv Rev Psychiatry 5:55–65, 1997

Blacklow RS, Broadhead WE, Weissman M, et al: Symptom-Driven Diagnostic System—Primary Care (SDDS-PC): a report of work in progress. Paper presented at the 16th Annual NIMH International Research Conference on Primary Mental Health Research: Concepts, Methods and Obstacles, Tysons Corner, VA, September 1992

Bolund C: Suicide and cancer, I: demographic and social characteristics of cancer patients who committed suicide in Sweden, 1973–1976. Journal of Psychosocial Oncology 3:17–30, 1985a

Bolund C: Suicide and cancer, II: medical and care factors in suicides by cancer patients in Sweden, 1973–1976. Journal of Psychosocial Oncology 3:31–52, 1985b

Broadhead WE, Blazer DG, George LK, et al: Depression, disability days and days lost from work in a prospective epidemiologic survey. JAMA 264:2524–2528, 1990

Brody DS, Thompson TL II, Larson DB, et al: Recognizing and managing depression in primary care. Gen Hosp Psychiatry 17:93–107, 1995

Brown JH, Henteleff P, Barakat S, et al: Is it normal for terminally ill patients to desire death? Am J Psychiatry 143:208–211, 1986

Burnam MA, Wells KB, Leake B, et al: Development of a brief screening instrument for detecting depressive disorders. Med Care 26:775–789, 1988

Butler RN, Lewis MI: Late-life depression: when and how to intervene. Geriatrics 50(8):44–55, 1995

Campbell PC: Suicide among cancer patients. Connecticut Health Bulletin 80:207–212, 1966

Carlson GA: More analysis of Eli Robins' data (letter). Am J Psychiatry 141:323, 1984

Carney SS, Rich CL, Burke PA: Suicide over 60: The San Diego Study. J Am Geriatr Soc 42:174–180, 1994

Chia BH: Suicide and the generation gap. Suicide Life Threat Behav 2:194–208, 1979

Chynoweth R: Suicide in the elderly. Crisis 2:106–116, 1981

Chynoweth R, Tonge JI, Armstrong J: Suicide in Brisbane—a retrospective psychosocial study. Aust N Z J Psychiatry 14:37–45, 1980

Clark DC: Suicide Among the Elderly. Final report to the AARP Andrus Foundation. AARP Andrus Foundation, Washington, DC, January 28, 1991

Colenda CC, Sherman FT: Managed Medicare: an overview for the primary care physician. Geriatrics 53(1):57–63, 1998

Colenda CC, Banazak D, Mickus M: Mental health services in managed care: quality questions remain. Geriatrics 53(8):49–63, 1998

Conwell Y: Suicide in elderly patients, in Diagnosis and Treatment of Depression in Late Life. Edited by Schneider LS, Reynolds CF, Lebowitz BD, et al. Washington, DC, American Psychiatric Press, 1994, pp 397–418

Conwell Y, Rotenberg M, Caine ED: Completed suicide at age 50 and over. J Am Geriatr Soc 38:640–644, 1990

Conwell Y, Caine ED, Flannery CJ, et al: Suicide and aging: psychological autopsy findings. Paper presented at the 144th annual meeting of the American Psychiatric Association. New Orleans, LA, May 1991

Coulehan JL, Schulberg HC, Block MR, et al: Depressive symptomatology and medical co-morbidity in a primary care clinic. Int J Psychiatry Med 20:335–347, 1990

Curran DK: Adolescent Suicidal Behavior. New York, Hemisphere, 1987

Darbonne AR: Suicide and age: a suicide note analysis. J Consult Clin Psychol 33:46–50, 1969

De Leo D, Rozzini R, Bernardini M, et al: Assessment of quality of life in the elderly assisted at home through a tele-check service. Quality of Life Research 1:367–374, 1992

De Leo D, Carollo G, Buono MD: Lower suicide rates associated with a tele-help/tele-check service for the elderly at home. Am J Psychiatry 152:632–634, 1995

Depression Guideline Panel: Depression in Primary Care, Vol 1: Detection and Diagnosis (AHCPR Publ No 93-0550; Clinical Practice Guideline No 5). Rockville, MD, U.S. Dept of Health and Human Services, Agency for Health Care Policy and Research, April 1993a

Depression Guideline Panel. Depression in Primary Care, Vol 2: Treatment of Major Depression (AHCPR Publ No 93-0551; Clinical Practice Guideline No 5). Rockville, MD, U.S. Dept of Health and Human Services, Agency for Health Care Policy and Research, April 1993b

Dew MA, Bromet EJ, Brent D, et al: A quantitative literature review of the effectiveness of suicide prevention centers. J Consult Clin Psychol 55:239–244, 1987

Dorpat TL, Ripley HS. A study of suicide in the Seattle area. Compr Psychiatry 1:349–359, 1960

Dorpat TL, Anderson WF, Ripley HS: The relationship of physical illness to suicide, in Suicidal Behaviors: Diagnosis and Management. Edited by Resnik HLP. Boston, MA, Little, Brown, 1968, pp 209–219

Draper B: Suicidal behavior in the elderly. Int J Geriatr Psychiatry 9:655–661, 1994

Eisdorfer C: Managed care and mental health services. Paper presented at the annual meeting of the American Society on Aging. Atlanta, GA, March 1995

Eisenberg L: Treating depression and anxiety in primary care. N Engl J Med 326:1080–1084, 1992

Farberow NL, Schneidman ES, Leonard CV: Suicide among general medical and surgical hospital patients with malignant neoplasms (Medical Bulletin 9). Washington, DC, Department of Medicine and Surgery, Veterans Administration, 1963

Felton BJ: The aged: settings, services and needs, in Reaching the Underserved: Mental Health Needs of Neglected Populations. Edited by Snowden LR. Beverly Hills, CA, Sage, 1982, pp 23–42

Filiberti A, Ripamonti C, Saita L, et al: Frequency of suicide in cancer at the National Cancer Institute of Milan over 1986–90 (letter). Ann Oncol 2:610, 1991

Fox BH, Stanek S, Boyd SC, et al: Suicide rates among cancer patients in Connecticut. J Chronic Dis 35:89–100, 1982

Frankish CJ: Crisis centers and their role in treatment: suicide prevention versus health promotion. Death Studies 18:327–339, 1994

Gatz M, Smyer MA: The mental health system and older adults in the 1990s. Am Psychol 47:741–751, 1992

German PS, Shapiro S, Skinner EA: Mental health of the elderly: use of health and mental health services. J Am Geriatr Soc 33:246–252, 1985

Goldberg D, Steele JJ, Johnson A, et al: Ability of primary care physicians to make accurate ratings of psychiatric symptoms. Arch Gen Psychiatry 39:829–833, 1982

Goldberg RJ: Integrated Behavioral Health Services With General Medical Care. Providence, RI, Manisses Communications Group, Inc., 1996

Greenberg PE, Stiglin LE, Finkelstein SN, et al: The economic burden of depression in 1990. J Clin Psychiatry 54:405–418, 1993

Heikkinen ME, Isometsa ET, Aro HM, et al: Age-related variation in recent life events preceding suicide. J Nerv Ment Dis 183:325–331, 1995

Hietanen P, Lonnqvist J: Cancer and suicide. Ann Oncol 2:219–223, 1991

Hoeper EW, Kessler LG, Nycz G, et al: The usefulness of screening for mental illness. Lancet 1:33–35, 1984

Isometsa ET, Aro HM, Henriksson MM, et al: Suicide in major depression in different treatment settings. J Clin Psychiatry 55:523–527, 1994a

Isometsa ET, Henriksson MM, Aro HM, et al: Suicide in major depression. Am J Psychiatry 151:530–536, 1994b

Jarvis Gk, Boldt M: Suicide in the later years. Essence 4:144–158, 1980

Johnson J, Weissman MM, Klerman GL: Service utilization and social morbidity associated with depressive symptoms in the community. JAMA 267:1478–1483, 1992

Jones JS, Stanley B, Mann JJ, et al: CSF 5-HIAA and HVA concentrations in elderly depressed patients who attempted suicide. Am J Psychiatry 147:1225–1227, 1990

Jorm AF: The epidemiology of depressive states in the elderly: implications for recognition, intervention, and prevention. Soc Psychiatry Psychiatr Epidemiol 30:53–59, 1995

Katon W, Schulberg H: Epidemiology of depression in primary care. Gen Hosp Psychiatry 14:237–247, 1992

Katon W, Berg AO, Robins AJ, et al: Depression: medical utilization and somatization. West J Med 144:564–568, 1986

Katon W, Von Korff M, Lin E, et al: Adequacy and duration of antidepressant treatment in primary care. Med Care 30:67–76, 1992

Kessler LB, Amick BC III, Thompson J: Factors influencing the diagnosis of mental disorder among primary care patients. Med Care 23:50–62, 1985a

Kessler LB, Cleary PD, Burke JD: Psychiatric disorders in primary care: results of a follow-up study. Arch Gen Psychiatry 42:583–587, 1985b

Kochanek KD, Hudson BL: Advance report of final mortality statistics, 1992. Monthly Vital Statistics Report 43:23, 1995

Kontaxakis VP, Christodoulou GN, Mavreas VG, et al: Attempted suicide in psychiatric outpatients with concurrent physical illness. Psychother Psychosom 50:201–206, 1988

Kwan AY-H: Suicide among the elderly: Hong Kong. Journal of Applied Gerontology 7:248–259, 1988

Lasoski MC: Reasons for low utilization of mental health services by the elderly, in Clinical Gerontology: A Guide to Assessment and Intervention. Edited by Brink TL. Binghamton, NY, Haworth, 1986, pp 1–18

Lester D, Beck AT: Age differences in patterns of attempted suicide. Omega 5:317–322, 1974

Lonnqvist J, Achte K: Follow-up study of the attempted suicides among the elderly in Helsinki in 1973–1979. Crisis 6:10–18, 1985

Louhivuori KA, Hakama M: Risk of suicide among cancer patients. Am J Epidemiol 109:59–65, 1979

Lyness JM, Conwell Y, Nelson JC: Suicide attempts in elderly psychiatric inpatients. J Am Geriatr Soc 40:320–324, 1992

Mackenzie TB, Popkin MK: Suicide in the medical patient. Int J Psychiatry Med 17:3–22, 1987

Mann JJ, Arango V: Integration of neurobiology and psychopathology in a unified model of suicidal behavior. J Clin Psychopharmacol 12(suppl):2S–7S, 1992

Manton KG, Blazer DG, Woodbury MA: Suicide in the middle age and later life: sex- and race-specific life table and cohort analyses. J Gerontol 42:219–227, 1987

Marshall JR, Burnett W, Brasure J: On precipitating factors: cancer as a cause of suicide. Suicide Life Threat Behav 13:15–27, 1983

McIntire MS, Angle CR: The taxonomy of suicide and self-poisoning: a pediatric perspective, in Self-Destructive Behavior in Children and Adolescents. Edited by Wells CF, Stuart IR. New York, Van Nostrand Reinhold, 1981, pp 224–249

McIntosh JL: Suicide: training and education needs with an emphasis on the elderly. Gerontology and Geriatrics Education 7:125–139, 1987

McIntosh JL: Suicide prevention in the elderly (age 65–99). Suicide Life Threat Behav 25:180–192, 1995a

McIntosh JL: USA Suicide: 1992 Official Final Data. Washington, DC, American Association of Suicidology, 1995b

McIntosh JL, Hubbard RW, Santos JF: Suicide among the elderly: a review of issues with case studies. Journal of Gerontology: Social Work 4:68–74, 1981

McIntosh JL, Santos JF, Hubbard RW, et al: Elder Suicide: Research, Theory and Treatment. Washington, DC, American Psychological Association, 1994

Murphy GE: The physician's responsibility for suicide: errors of omission. Ann Intern Med 82:305–309, 1975

Neimeyer RA, Pfeiffer AM: Evaluation of suicide intervention effectiveness. Death Studies 18:131–166, 1994

Nielsen AC, Williams TA: Depression in ambulatory medical patients: prevalence by self-report questionnaire and recognition by nonpsychiatric physicians. Arch Gen Psychiatry 37:999–1004, 1980

Nieto E, Vieta E, Lazaro L, et al: Serious suicide attempts in the elderly. Psychopathology 25:183–188, 1992

Ormel J, Koeter MWJ, van den Brink W, et al: Recognition, management and the course of anxiety and depression in general practice. Arch Gen Psychiatry 48:700–706, 1991

Osgood NJ: Suicide in the Elderly. Rockville, MD, Aspen, 1985

Osgood NJ: Prevention of suicide in the elderly. J Geriatr Psychiatry 24:293–306, 1991

Osgood NJ, Brant BA: Suicidal behavior in long-term care facilities. Suicide Life Threat Behav 20:113–122, 1990

Pandey GN, Pandey SC, Dwivedi Y, et al: Platelet serotonin-2A receptors: a potential biologic marker for suicidal behavior. Am J Psychiatry 152:850–855, 1995

Parkin D, Stengel E: Incidence of suicidal attempts in an urban community. BMJ 2:133–138, 1965

Perez EL, Blouin J: Psychiatric emergency consultations to elderly patients in a Canadian general hospital. J Am Geriatr Soc 34:91–94, 1986

Physician Payment Review Commission: Revising the method for determining Medicare capitated payments (chapter 3). Annual Report to Congress 1997, Washington, DC, 1997, pp 53–75

Pollinger-Haas A, Hendin H: Suicide among older people: projections for the future. Suicide Life Threat Behav 13:147–154, 1983

Pratt CC, Schmall VL, Wilson W, et al: A model community education program on depression and suicide in later life. Gerontologist 31:692–695, 1991

Rabins PV: Prevention of mental disorder in the elderly: current perspectives and future prospects. J Am Geriatr Soc 40:727–733, 1992

Redick RW, Taube CA: Demography of mental health care of the aged, in Handbook of Mental Health and Aging. Edited by Birren JE, Sloane RB. Englewood Cliffs, NJ, Prentice-Hall, 1980, pp 57–71

Regier DA, Goldberg ID, Taube CA: The de facto US mental health services system. Arch Gen Psychiatry 35:685–693, 1978

Rice DP, Kelman S, Miller LS, et al: The Economic Costs of Alcohol and Drug Abuse and Mental Illness. San Francisco, University of California, Institute for Health and Aging, 1990

Rich CL, Warsradt GM, Nemiroff RA, et al: Suicide, stressors and the life cycle. Am J Psychiatry 148:524–527, 1991

Robins E: The Final Months: A Study of the Lives of 134 Persons Who Committed Suicide. Oxford, UK, Oxford University Press, 1981

Robins E, Murphy GE, Wilkinson RH, et al: Some clinical considerations in the prevention of suicide based on a study of 134 successful suicides. Am J Public Health 48:888–899, 1959

Rodin G, Voshart K: Depressive symptoms and functional impairment in the medically ill. Gen Hosp Psychiatry 9:251–258, 1987

Rogers WH, Wells KB, Meredith LS, et al: Outcomes for adult outpatients with depression under prepaid or fee-for-service financing. Arch Gen Psychiatry 50:517–525, 1993

Rutz L, Von Knorring L, Walinder J: Frequency of suicide on Gotland after systematic postgraduate education of general practitioners. Acta Psychiatr Scand 80:151–154, 1989

Sainsbury P: Suicide in London (Maudsley Monographs No 1). London, Chapman & Hall, 1955

Sainsbury P: Suicide in middle and later years, in Aging Around the World: Medical and Clinical Aspects of Aging. Edited by Blumenthal HT. New York, Columbia University Press, 1962, pp 97–105

Sainsbury P: Social and epidemiological aspects of suicide with special references to the aged, in Process of Aging: Social and Psychological Perspectives. Edited by Williams RH, Tibbitts C, Donahue W. New York, Atherton Press, 1963, pp 153–175

Schwab JJ, Bialow M, Brown JM, et al: Diagnosing depression in medical inpatients. Ann Intern Med 67:695–707, 1967

Seller RH, Blascovich J, Lenkei E: Influence of stereotypes in the diagnosis of depression by family practice residents. J Fam Pract 12:849–854, 1981

Sendbuehler JM, Goldstein S: Attempted suicide among the aged. J Am Geriatr Soc 25:244–248, 1977

Shasha M, Lyons JS, O'Mahoney MT, et al: Serotonin reuptake inhibitors and the adequacy of antidepressant therapy. Int J Psychiatry Med 27:83–92, 1997

Shea D: Economic and financial issues in mental health and aging. Public Policy Aging Report 9(1):7–12, 1998

Sheikh JI, Yesavage JA: Geriatric Depression Scale (GDS): recent evidence and development of a shorter version, in Clinical Gerontology: A Guide to Assessment and Intervention. Edited by Brink TL. Binghamton, NY, Haworth, 1986, pp 165–173

Sheperd M, Cooper AG, Brown AC, et al: Psychiatric Illness in General Practice. New York, Oxford University Press, 1966

Sherman J: Medicare's Mental Health Benefits: Coverage, Utilization and Expenditures. Washington, DC, AARP Public Policy Institute, 1992

Skodol AE, Schwartz S, Dohrenwend BP, et al: Minor depression in a cohort of young adults in Israel. Arch Gen Psychiatry 51:542–551, 1994

Stenager EN, Stenager E: Suicide and patients with neurologic diseases: methodologic problems. Arch Neurol 49:1296–1303, 1992

Stenback A: Depression and suicidal behavior in old age, in Handbook of Mental Health and Aging. Edited by Birren JE, Sloane RB. Englewood Cliffs, NJ, Prentice-Hall, 1980, pp 616–652

Tarnopolsky A, Hand DJ, McLean EK, et al: Validity and uses of a screening questionnaire (GHQ) in the community. Br J Psychiatry 134:508–515, 1979

van Praag HM: Biological suicide research: outcome and limitations. Biol Psychiatry 21:1305–1323, 1986

Ware JE, Bayliss MS, Rogers WH, et al: Differences in 4-year health outcomes for elderly and poor, chronically ill patients treated in HMO and fee-for-service systems. JAMA 276:1039–1047, 1996

Wells KB: Depression as a Tracer Condition for the National Study of Medical Care Outcomes: Background Review (Publ R-3292-RWJ/HJK). Santa Monica, CA, The RAND Corporation, 1985

Wells KB, Manning WG, Benjamin B: Use of outpatient mental health services in HMO and fee-for-service plans: results from a randomized controlled trial. Health Serv Res 21:453–474, 1986a

Wells KB, Manning WG, Duan N, et al: Use of outpatient mental health services by a general population with health insurance coverage. Hospital and Community Psychiatry 37:1119–1125, 1986b

Wells KB, Hays RD, Burnam MA, et al: Detection of depressive disorder for patients receiving prepaid or fee-for-service care: results from the Medical Outcomes Study. JAMA 262:3298–3302, 1989a

Wells KB, Stewart A, Hays RD, et al: The functioning and well-being of depressed patients: results of the Medical Outcomes Study. JAMA 262:914–919, 1989b

Wells KB, Katon W, Rogers WH, et al: Use of minor tranquilizers and antidepressant medications by depressed outpatients: results from the Medical Outcomes Study. Am J Psychiatry 151:694–700, 1994

Whitlock FA: Suicide, cancer and depression. Br J Psychiatry 132:269–274, 1978

Whitlock FA: Suicide and physical illness, in Suicide. Edited by Roy A. Baltimore, MD, Williams & Wilkins, 1986, pp 151–170

Williams JBW, Spitzer RL: PRIME-MD: a new system for the evaluation of mental disorders in primary care. Paper presented at the 16th Annual NIMH International Research Conference on Primary Mental Health Research: Concepts, Methods and Obstacles. Tysons Corner, VA, September 1992

Winchel RM, Stanley B, Stanley M: Biochemical aspects of suicide, in Suicide Over the Life Cycle: Risk Factors, Assessment, and Treatment of Suicidal Patients. Edited by Blumenthal SJ, Kupfer DJ. Washington, DC, American Psychiatric Press, 1990, pp 97–126

Zimmerman M, Coryell W: The Inventory to Diagnose Depression (IDD): a self-report scale to diagnose major depressive disorder. J Consult Clin Psychol 55:55–59, 1987

Zung WWK: A self-rating depression scale. Arch Gen Psychiatry 12:63–70, 1965

CHAPTER 6

Substance Abuse and Suicidal Behavior in Managed Care

Richard Caplan, M.S.W., M.P.H.

Substance abuse, so often a factor in parasuicidal and suicidal behavior, requires special attention during the process of suicide assessment, treatment planning, and delivery of care. In this chapter, I discuss issues that affect the care of suicidal substance abusers, with emphasis on those enrolled in managed care systems. The term *managed care*, as used here, embraces a wide variety of health care delivery systems that share administrative and structural elements such as preauthorization of care, utilization management, case management, and a limited benefit design. I review the relationship between substance abuse and suicidality, address the concerns that arise during different stages of care, and describe how a managed care system can facilitate successful care with specific attention to the risk of suicidal behavior. While the focus here is on managed care systems, many of the issues discussed are also relevant to care in other systems of care.

Substance Abuse and Suicidality

Among the approximately 30,000 completed suicides that occur annually in the United States, between 20% and 35% of completers had a history of alcohol abuse or were drinking shortly before their suicides (Secretary of Health and Human Services 1990). Suicide attempts are 8–14 times as frequent as completed suicides (Petronis et al. 1990) and are far more frequent among substance abusers than in the general population. Fifteen percent of alcoholic men and 40% of alcoholic women, compared with 2.9% of the general population (National Committee for Injury Prevention and Control 1990), are reported to have attempted suicide (Gomberg 1989; Kolozsi 1990). Suicide attempts by substance abusers are more lethal, too.

One of the key differences between those who attempt and those who complete suicide is the presence of substance abuse (National Center for Health Statistics 1991). The risk that an attempt will lead to a completed suicide is estimated to be seven times greater among those with alcohol use disorders compared with those without such disorders (Myers et al. 1984; Petronis et al. 1990). In one study, the very high suicide completion rate of 25% was found among the known alcoholic or drug-addicted individuals who attempted suicide (Miller et al. 1991).

Fully 70% of adolescent suicide attempts may be complicated by drug and alcohol abuse and dependence (Miller et al. 1991). In one study, substance abuse was the most frequent characteristic of the adolescents who attempted suicide (Miller et al. 1991). In view of such alarming data, the National Institute of Mental Health has designated alcohol abuse as one of the greatest risk factors for a suicide attempt in the adolescent population (National Committee for Injury Prevention and Control 1990).

Far less is known about the effect that other recreational substances have on suicide attempts or completions. Substances other than alcohol may be less frequently used as a suicide method by those individuals addicted to those substances. For example, although the prevalence of suicide attempts among individuals addicted to opioids is estimated to be between 8% and 17% (Krausz et al. 1996), heroin overdose in and of itself is considered a rare suicide method (Gottschalk et al. 1979). Studies on cocaine (Clark and Sperry 1988) suggest that cocaine itself is not frequently the vehicle for suicidal behavior but that the "crash" associated with cocaine withdrawal may stimulate or exacerbate suicidal impulses. The greater prevalence of benzodiazepine use among women has been suggested to be one of the factors responsible for women's higher rate of suicide attempts. Since benzodiazepines are so often used in combination with alcohol or other drugs, however, it is difficult to determine whether benzodiazepine overdoses imply prior dependency, abuse, or merely use of these drugs as a means for suicide (Michel et al. 1994). The relationship of suicide to tobacco use has been explored preliminarily. There is a suggestion that the use of cigarettes, perhaps as a correlate of other psychiatric and substance abuse problems, may be a marker for greater suicide risk (Hemenway et al. 1993).

Alcohol and Suicidal Behavior

Although no unitary mechanism has been established to explain the relationship between substance abuse and suicide, alcohol appears to increase suicide risk in a variety of clinically understandable ways. It impairs *judgment,* affecting perception and interpretation of surrounding circumstances and events in a way that may adversely influence a person's choice of actions. It counteracts appropriate *inhibition,* impairing ability to forego potentially dangerous or self-destructive actions in favor of safer alternative behaviors. It increases *depression* after a brief initial period of excitation and can exacerbate a mood disturbance already present, increasing the likelihood of suicidal ideation or behavior (National Committee for Injury Prevention and Control 1990). Excessive alcohol use and drug use also correlate with *social isolation.* The waning of relationships other than those associated with substance use may mean limited emotional supports during times of crisis. Family, friends, and co-workers who are part of an existing support network may become increasingly unavailable as a person's substance use progresses. Finally, alcoholic individuals are far more likely than the general population to carry a diagnosis of *antisocial personality disorder,* which in itself is a strong risk factor for suicide attempts (Helzer and Pryzbeck 1988).

Other Drugs and Suicidal Behavior

For the cocaine-dependent substance abuser, the time of highest suicide risk is during the "crash" phase of withdrawal, often the morning after a night of intense abuse. At this time, the patient is exhausted, depleted, and often filled with shame and guilt. This is the moment of greatest danger for self-harm. The suicidal feelings of a cocaine abuser, however, are often transient experiences that subside dramatically after a meal and some sleep. The formerly suicidal cocaine abuser, after a rest, may transform into a more cooperative individual, for the moment less intent on self-destruction.

Abusers of heroin and other opiates devote enormous energy to avoiding the unpleasant consequences of drug withdrawal. An opiate abuser who reaches the clinician's office, therefore, is likely to be already in great distress, experiencing the discomfort of a withdrawal made necessary by lack of funds or unavailability of drugs. Such an individual's primary concern is relief from physical discomfort, nausea, or pain. Some patients in active opiate withdrawal express suicidal or other dangerous intentions as part of an effort to acquire more drugs. It is often best to avoid putting closure on a diagnostic formulation of such a patient until after a treatment protocol for reducing withdrawal symptoms has begun. Once symptomatic relief has been provided with medication, an opiate abuser may become more communicative and cooperative.

Unlike users of substances with more extreme and rapid effects, marijuana users ease into their dependence more gradually. As involvement with marijuana increasingly absorbs the abuser, normal tasks of development and socialization may be increasingly neglected. Marijuana users may dull internal conflict with intoxication that conceals the development of suicidal feelings and defers the imminence of suicidal actions. The extended duration of marijuana effects accounts for the infrequency and mildness of withdrawal symptoms.

Some substance abusers pursue a pattern of indiscriminate polysubstance ingestion, swallowing any available prescribed or illicit pills alone or in combination. Some easily obtained combinations—for example, fluoxetine and dextromethorphan—can result in intense interactive effects. These indiscriminate polysubstance users are often the most difficult to rehabilitate, and their risk for self-harm is among the most lethal. When presenting for acute treatment, such abusers may actually be unable to determine what pills they have ingested. Comorbid psychiatric illnesses, including not only personality disturbances but also mood, anxiety, or psychotic disorders, are often present.

Suicidal Substance Abusers in Managed Care

By the end of 1995, 161 million Americans, accounting for more then 60% of the population, were enrolled in some form of managed health care. The domination of mental health and substance abuse treatment by managed care has been equally rapid. By the end of 1995, managed care systems controlled the mental health and substance abuse benefits of nearly 142 million people in both public and private sectors (Edmunds et al. 1997).

Though the quality of care delivered by such systems remains a subject of active public debate, the components of managed care have the potential for improving the effectiveness of treatment of substance abusers. While acknowledging the potential problems in managed care, I discuss here ways in which elements of managed care could improve the preventive care, acute assessment and stabilization, follow-up, and rehabilitative care of substance abusers under optimal circumstances. The examples used to illustrate this discussion are composite cases that draw on clinical experience but disguise patients' identifying characteristics in order to preserve their anonymity.

Substance abuse treatment comprises a series of stages. Primary prevention requires intervention prior to actual substance abuse, and secondary prevention implies the use of interventions that decrease the morbidity of ongoing substance abuse. Acute assessment and stabilization become necessary when intoxication impairs a person's capacity to function appropriately or to remain safe from the danger of harm to self or others. Reassessment, once intoxication has cleared, allows determination of a more reliable diagnostic formulation and facilitates treatment planning. Even when further episodes of acute assessment and stabilization are likely to be required as a result of relapses, there is a very important role for rehabilitation interventions in the follow-up care of substance abusers. Rehabilitative treatment focuses on acquisition of behavioral skills to be used in the maintenance of sobriety, the repair of damaged relationships, and the improvement of impaired functions.

Preventive Care

Substance abuse treatment is, despite clinicians' and patients' fears to the contrary, an effective means of reducing substance abuse and secondary morbidity (Gerstein et al. 1992; McLellan et al. 1992, 1994). The earlier substance abuse is diagnosed, the greater the likelihood of a successful outcome of treatment (Zwick and Bermon 1992).

Managed systems of care are in many ways uniquely positioned to promote the early identification of substance abusers. Systems that effectively integrate mental health/substance abuse services with primary care can implement systems for the early identification of substance abusers and facilitate their referral into specialty care venues by training primary care clinicians in assessment and diagnosis. Once a substance abuser is identified, substance abuse specialists can then work with primary care clinicians or other mental health personnel to provide ongoing support and consultation.

Advanced information systems, made necessary by the administrative needs of large systems for the provision of care, also make conceivable the systematic identification of patients who use large amounts of health care, present medical symptoms or findings typically associated with substance abuse, or receive excessive or duplicate abusable prescriptions. In time, health care systems may develop systems for the automatic early identification of individuals at risk or actively engaged in substance abuse much the way credit card companies already detect and query customers whose financial activities exceed expected levels.

Acute Assessment and Stabilization

Assessment begins the moment a patient presents for care. Stabilization involves attention to acute medical needs that require urgent care. Initial assessment may occur through a phone contact or visit to an outpatient or emergency room clinician. Medical stabilization is most usually handled in an emergency medical or detoxification setting, though some partial hospitalization or inpatient psychiatric programs are able to offer limited stabilization services.

When alcohol or drugs are present during a suicide assessment, an immediate need is to determine the patient's type and degree of intoxication. The clinician must determine how intoxication will affect the validity of further assessment and must decide, often immediately, whether emergency medical intervention is required. When there is doubt regarding the patient's safety, more stringent measures should be chosen as a default because survival may be in jeopardy.

Some substance users seek help voluntarily, while others are forced to find medical attention when drugs of abuse become unobtainable or when the medical consequences of intoxication or withdrawal become intolerable. Some seek help on their own initiative, while others are pressured to get help by concerned significant others, law enforcement personnel, or employers. During the initial assessment and stabilization phase of treatment, it is common for suicidal thoughts and behaviors to come to light. Assessing the suicide risk of an unfamiliar and intoxicated person is very unreliable, but an initial judgment of dangerousness must always be made nonetheless and can be regarded as a point of reference for comparison during subsequent reassessments.

As discussed in greater detail in Chapter 1 of this volume, any suicide risk assessment must address at least the patient's demographic risk factors, previous self-destructive behaviors, current stressors and supports, and degree of lethality and accessibility associated with current suicidal impulses, thoughts, or plans. In addition, the clinician must attempt an accurate and thorough assessment of substance use, including recent drug abuse patterns, current and past treatments, and any history of current or prior self-destructive behaviors associated with substance abuse.

The intoxicated patient often is incapable or unwilling to provide sufficient information. Furthermore, the mental status of an intoxicated patient is in flux and may change dramatically as drug effects subside. For these reasons, it may be necessary to detain a possibly suicidal patient until sobriety allows more reliable assessment. In the meantime, existing medical and psychiatric records and information from other informants who are familiar with the patient can be of vital importance (American Psychiatric Association 1995).

Toxicology and other diagnostic studies are routinely considered and often a necessity in assessing an acutely suicidal substance abuser. Often it is through such studies that the use of undisclosed substances or ingestion of poisons is recognized. Quantitative blood levels can also facilitate the diagnostic and treatment planning process in overdose emergencies that require medical interventions such as dialysis. When specific drugs or medications included in the overdose are known, the laboratory can be alerted to include these in their testing procedures, since not all recreationally abused drugs are included in the routine toxic screen panels. Other blood tests, X rays, or electrocardiography may be necessary to assess medical safety or identify life-threatening consequences of substance abuse or concurrent disorders. The medically unstable patient—for example, the profoundly intoxicated individual—may require temporary transfer to a medical unit for monitoring of vital signs or more intensive medical care.

The use of auxiliary informants should be handled with respect for the patient's confidentiality, but the presence of a life-threatening emergency justifies a clinician's effort to seek additional information even without a patient's specific consent. Indeed, when grave danger may threaten a patient's survival, it is far more risky to preserve confidentiality than to divulge what is necessary in order to gather data from additional informants in order to guide potentially life-saving treatment. Significant others or friends who brought the patient to the emergency room, for example, may be able to contribute valuable insights and information that will improve the patient's assessment and stabilization.

As discussed in greater depth in Appendix A of this volume, suicidal behavior or ideation may serve many goals beyond merely ending life. Sometimes the most important goals, objectives of which even the patient remains only partially aware, must be inferred during careful assessment. Suicidality, for example, can represent a covert request for additional or continued care, an expression of anger at unfulfilled treatment expectations, a desperate measure for avoiding painful emotional experience, or a last-ditch response to life's immediate pressures when all available resources have been exhausted.

Especially among recidivists, suicidal behavior may serve as a plea for further care. Substance abusers who have been repeatedly admitted for observation or detoxification may fear that only the threat of dangerous behavior will open the door to further resources. Such a patient learns that the words "suicide" or "homicide" evoke a rapid clinical response. Clinicians faced with the responsibility of assessing such a patient must be careful not to communicate rejection, which will often lead the patient to escalate his or her threats to a more strident level.

Case Example

The emergency room psychiatric resident on call was asked to evaluate Arnold, a 68-year-old intoxicated man who threatened to kill himself if not admitted to the hospital. Arnold admitted to recent abuse of codeine, but denied use of drugs capable of inducing life-threatening withdrawal states. Once he was medically cleared and assessed to be at low risk of dangerous behavior, he was asked to make an appointment the following day in the outpatient clinic. On his way out the door, he said angrily, "If I have to hurt myself for you to take me seriously, I will!" Minutes later, he returned with deep self-inflicted wrist lacerations that led to his admission.

Substance-abusing individuals with comorbid personality disorders may demonstrate hostile transferential feelings toward their caregivers through self-injurious behaviors. The patient who has formed a dependent attachment to a health care provider may encounter disturbing, regressive longings to be cared for and freed of life's responsibilities. The perceived promise of care and protection arouses expectations in some that cannot be met within the realistic limitations of a health care system. When the inevitable disappointment arrives, suicidal behavior may result. The risk for such behavior is amplified when alcohol or other drugs disinhibit the patient's usual level of self-restraint. Faced with such a patient, health care providers must be especially careful to avoid promising what they cannot provide.

Case Example

Maryanne, a 19-year-old chronically suicidal adolescent, had a history of sexual abuse, eating disorders, and cocaine dependence. Her initial involvement with the mental health department of an health maintenance organization (HMO) ushered in several months of hopefulness and happiness, as she experienced consistent response to her needs and empathy with her suffering. During the maternity leave of one of her clinicians, she felt abandoned and betrayed. She expressed her outrage by resuming her cocaine abuse, concluding a 2-week binge with a serious overdose of her mother's medications.

Some individuals with depression or anxiety disorders may turn to substances to relieve their symptoms. In these patients, suicidal behavior may represent a self-medicating attempt to avoid suffering. Such people typically lack the developed capacity to endure and work through the pain of psychic or physical distress. The clinician faced with such an individual must respect the protective power of denial, a defense that can keep self-destructive feelings at bay through avoidance of the intolerable experience of intense affect. Even pleasurable feelings may be regarded as a threat, and some patients may fear that their feelings can literally kill them—a fear unfortunately borne out when suicide is the result.

Case Example

Gail, a 42-year-old alcoholic woman, was 18 months into her sobriety when she met a man and quickly became sexually intimate. Since her entire sobriety until that point had been experienced in isolation, her new involvement evoked intense feelings. She experienced intolerable suicidal ideation and had to be hospitalized. Her fear of intimacy and, consequently, risk of abandonment were so great and her skills to deal with these feelings were so limited that she seriously considered dying to be more tolerable than working through her feelings.

Suicide, for some, serves as a final option for avoiding chronic pain, humiliation, poverty, or other intolerable life circumstances. Once all other possibilities are apparently exhausted, the risk of suicide escalates. People with limited internal or external resources may reach the decision to attempt suicide sooner than others with more options. Intoxication adds to the lethality of these patients' choices by limiting the ability to assess realistic choices. The clinician who assesses a patient in this type of scenario may be able to protect the patient by identifying overlooked alternative behaviors.

Case Example

Susan, a 45-year-old unattached schoolteacher, had struggled with chronic marijuana use, alcohol abuse, and the pain of progressive arthritis since she was an adolescent. She lived an isolated life, with no friends and a toxic family. When her absenteeism resulted in unwillingness of her school district to renew her contract, she saw no other job possibilities. She had enough money to stay in her apartment for another month or two, after which she would be homeless without a source of income. Although Susan was able to stop her use of marijuana and moderate her alcohol use, she looked ahead at what she perceived to be the inexorable approach of poverty and homelessness and concluded that suicide was her only option.

As discussed more broadly in Chapter 2 of this volume with respect to all suicidal patients, managed care systems can facilitate assessment of the suicidal patient in a variety of ways. First, the availability of a designated central screening facility (often reached through a toll-free phone number) can provide knowledgeable and immediate access to care. Ideally, the clinician at the other end of the line will know what questions to ask in order to assess the dangerousness of the situation. When needed, an ambulance or rescue team can be immediately dispatched. For less acute needs, the telephone screener (not a "hot line" for counseling, but rather the system for accessing care) can provide a list of clinicians who are able to provide further evaluation and treatment. In a network system, referral to a geographically convenient provider should be possible. When phone screeners are uncertain as to the serious of a caller's condition, the availability of a crisis service, with holding capacity, offers the opportunity to gain additional clinical information in a face-to-face assessment.

The comprehensive information systems employed by many managed care organizations may allow evaluating clinicians to obtain access to information about the patient's past or current treatment contacts. This serves the patient's needs better by facilitating communication with involved caregivers—an important aspect of assessment that can be made more difficult when intoxication renders the patient uncooperative or unresponsive. Comprehensive information systems also help clinicians remain aware of concurrent medical problems or medications that might complicate the effects of intoxication or withdrawal. The interrelationships between levels of care within a managed system facilitate arrangement of follow-up care once the patient is stabilized and reassessed.

In some communities, the aggressive marketing of managed care programs has produced a regrettable drawback by fostering unrealistic expectations of care. When, for example, a patient seeks treatment at a specific facility that is not affiliated with the managed care network, authorization of treatment may not be forthcoming. A frustration-intolerant substance-abusing individual may react with rage and a sense of abandonment rather than accept referral to a less desired institution within the network of covered providers. When refusal of a specific request is received by an individual with a history of being neglected by a dysfunctional family, it may take skillful negotiation to convince the patient that the available care is an appropriate alternative. Further disappointments may occur when a patient's allotted visits for a calendar year run out, requiring an increased expenditure on the patient's part in order to continue treatment. The clinician's responsibilities in such situations are discussed in Chapter 8 of this volume, while the process of appeal is reviewed in Chapter 2 and in Appendix B.

Reassessment

Usually, the assessing clinician must decide at an early stage whether to focus a patient's further treatment more predominantly on substance abuse or on psychiatric issues. Depressive symptoms secondary to alcohol abuse may well subside after even a day or two of abstinence and observation (Brown and Schuckit 1988; DeSoto et al. 1989; Schuckit 1986), whereas patients whose depression is primary may look even more distressed once the intoxication has cleared. This is one means by which appropriate follow-up can be determined relatively quickly.

When intoxication and depressive or anxiety symptoms clear rapidly, the clinician's challenge may include convincing the patient that the suicidal behavior was meaningful and a signal that acute or follow-up psychiatric treatment is indicated. The patient may even be partially or wholly amnestic for the behaviors that led to assessment. When patients' preexisting tendency to deny or excuse their actions is facilitated by intoxication, the likelihood of treatment compliance may be greatly reduced. Patients with this behavior pattern often end up repetitively harming themselves.

During reassessment, family members, employers, partners, friends, or other significant persons connected with the patient can be invited to provide further information. At this point, however, the situation may not be life-threatening and the patient's right to confidentiality would then need to be respected by obtaining appropriate permission for these contacts.

During reassessment, it is valuable to learn more about the patient from a now-sober informant. Have there been previous similar episodes? Is the current behavior part of an escalating pattern? What has helped in the past? Has the patient followed up with past treatment recommendations?

Reassessment, because it precedes a decision about disposition, can be an even more challenging task than initial assessment and stabilization. The managed care system that makes available more extensive information from past episodes and other care providers facilitates this stage of treatment. Many managed care systems maintain a set of treatment protocols, too, that help guide clinicians' choices during reassessment by specifying the clinical characteristics that determine admission to various levels of subsequent care.

When extended observation is necessary before appropriate disposition can be securely decided, managed care networks may be at an advantage over many other systems of care. The hospital emergency room staff, eager to free space for the next patient, may attempt to accelerate discharge of an intoxicated patient. A holding bed in a managed care crisis clinic, by contrast, serves the needs of both patient and provider by extending observation, thereby potentially avoiding an unnecessary admission to a more intensive (and expensive) level of care. Because coverage of a large number of "lives" allows economy of scale, a managed care system may include a round-the-clock crisis service staffed with clinicians who have expertise in both substance abuse and psychiatry and access to observation/holding beds that facilitate the process of reassessment.

Case Examples *(continued)*

Once Arnold's lacerations were sutured, he was admitted to an observation bed. With additional information obtained from Arnold and his wife, who was reached by telephone, the crisis clinician became concerned about the presence of a chronic and untreated mood disorder.

Maryanne's overdose required immediate intensive medical care. Once stabilized, she continued to experience suicidal urges and expressed a sense of futility at having failed in her attempt to end her life.

Gail was quickly assessed to be sober and was congratulated for maintaining her resolve not to drink even in the face of such a severe stressor. Her most immediate preoccupation was what her new boyfriend would do when he learned of her crisis.

Susan revealed her despair and pain in the crisis clinic and expressed her wish to find a way to continue living and to deal with her difficulties. Her acute suicidal urges quickly subsided once she regained hope of finding other ways to cope.

Follow-Up Care

Once reassessed by a clinician in a face-to-face interview, the patient is ready for referral to the next phase of care. Options at this point include an additional stay in the observation area, referral for detoxification and/or inpatient psychiatric treatment, attendance at an intensive outpatient setting such as a day or evening treatment program, or transfer back to a preexisting medical or substance abuse/mental health clinician and established support system.

While it is recognized that some patients will feel unfairly constrained by limitations that may be imposed on their treatment choices, it is nonetheless true that managed care systems with an organized approach to care may have much to offer the suicidal substance abuser seeking follow-up care. Quality care can be facilitated by the availability of a continuum of services, coordination of care providers, a flexible and responsive benefit structure, and the option of using a case manager. These attributes are often part of a managed care system.

By contracting with or running centralized programs filled by referrals from a surrounding network of providers, many managed care systems are able to provide their members with a continuum of care that is both accessible and convenient. Partial hospital or day programs provide supervision for patients who are too unstable to work or to remain at home unsupervised during business hours. For patients who are able to return to work but still unsteady in sobriety, an evening program can provide support during hours that would otherwise be a time of risk for relapse of substance abuse.

Patients with ambivalence about follow-up are sometimes unnecessarily lost to treatment when transfer between programs is handled too loosely. In many managed care systems, coordination of outpatient providers with more intensive programs is an expected aspect of treatment. Discharge from the holding bed or detoxification unit, for example, should include arrangement of a follow-up appointment with the intensive outpatient program or other outpatient provider.

Flexible options for the use of benefits facilitate transfer of patients between levels of care. A program that allows the exchange of one inpatient care day for two partial hospital days, for example, both eases the patient's access to appropriate care and supports the use of the least restrictive appropriate setting for care. Similar exchanges between individual and group treatment sessions may offer patients the option of attending a support group for an extended period of time. Clear, thoughtful criteria should be used to determine which levels of treatment will be made available to patients by spelling out the criteria for admission to each level or program.

When case management services are accessed, managed care providers can follow their patients as they move across several levels of care. Managed care's philosophy of case management is one of its most significant contributions to the delivery of health care. By designating a mental health/substance abuse clinician to follow the patient's care, the managed care system conceptualizes treatment within a disease management model (i.e., prevention, intervention, management, and follow-up) instead of as a string of fragmented episodes of crisis and acute care. The case manager's job is to stay with the patient across each level of care, to coordinate the referrals, and to confirm attendance. If the patient drops out of a program or attends only sporadically, the case manager can attempt to reengage the patient in treatment. At each phase of treatment, the patient with a case manager can make use of that consistent presence to advocate for or to encourage and explain aspects of treatment. Eventually, the case manager will reconnect the patient with preexisting outpatient clinicians or knit together a new team of clinicians to address continuing medical and substance abuse concerns.

Case Examples *(continued)*

Arnold was admitted to a day hospital that specialized in the treatment of dually diagnosed patients. Once he was started on an antidepressant and encouraged to attend 12-Step groups, his willingness to cooperate with treatment improved.

When Maryanne became medically stable, she was transferred to an inpatient psychiatric unit that provided care in a nonregressive and highly structured program. The inpatient program helped her transition back to outpatient care with her former psychotherapist while educating her about emergency resources, such as a suicide hotline for use during future crises. Her cocaine use diminished as she learned more about the potential consequences of this behavior. She also began to attend a dialectical behavior therapy–oriented group that included other young women with histories of sexual abuse.

Gail was discharged from the crisis clinic with a follow-up referral for individual psychotherapy. She reconnected with her AA sponsor and attended meetings more frequently in the subsequent weeks. Eventually, as her intimate relationship continued, she found it helpful to receive couples counseling with her new partner.

Susan was assigned a case manager who helped her access emergency financial support and obtain medical treatment for her arthritis. Although marijuana and alcohol had dulled her physical and emotional pains, she was helped to find other means for achieving relief.

Rehabilitation

Treatment does not end with the resolution of one substance abuse crisis. Instead, the process of recovery and rehabilitation often extends over a period of years. Public and professional critics have accused managed care systems of limiting care for chronic mental health and substance abuse conditions. The primary concerns expressed are that such systems of care either lack sufficient benefits or restrict access to substance abuse treatment. While such criticisms await further study, we can already assert that for managed care to truly provide good care for mental health or substance abuse issues, there must be a flexible benefit based on clinical criteria so that ongoing supportive treatments, including rehabilitation-oriented treatments, will remain available for patients as part of a total treatment plan. To skimp on care at this stage of treatment would indeed be shortsighted, increasing the likelihood of relapse and the need for more acute care.

Teaching, planning, supervising, and engaging the patient in a process of care form the heart of the rehabilitation phase of treatment. These elements of treatment are introduced as soon as the patient becomes sober and attentive. Over time, these aspects of treatment take center stage.

Engagement of significant others, including friends, partners, families, employers, and other supports, is an important aspect of rehabilitation. Common wisdom dictates that if you cannot get the substance abuser to get healthier, you work on getting the support system healthier. This puts further pressure on the patient to act in healthier ways or face clear, specific, undesirable contingencies.

Much like schizophrenia, alcoholism or substance abuse is a chronic debilitating condition that will most often worsen if not treated. Substance abusers are prone to relapse if they are not following their treatment plan. One way managed care has made possible the ongoing care of such patients is to provide a "chronic care" benefit. This allows substance abusers the chance to remain in recovery groups as long as needed. This is actually a very practical and cost-effective way of managing a chronic, high-risk population.

The Perils of Sobriety

One of the more dangerous things that can happen to a sober substance abuser is to feel "good." People in early recovery have no idea what "good" feels like and are quite fearful of it. For many patients who were raised in chaotic and dysfunctional family environments, "good" feelings may be so unfamiliar and therefore uncomfortable that their presence is not well tolerated. If another crisis does not arrive soon, these patients might semiconsciously precipitate one as a means of experiencing more familiar, and therefore more tolerable, feelings of dysphoria, anxiety, anger, or fear.

It is important that clinicians remain watchful when a patient reports feeling good during an early stage of recovery. Typical managed care "chronic care" benefits and the ability to follow patients over a long period of time allow for managed care providers to stay involved in a patient's life at least for that first full year of sobriety. Managed care systems should also have the ability to recruit and coordinate nutritional, dental, and other specialty care that the patient may find useful as he or she recovers from dependence on substances.

No discussion of suicidality and substance abuse would be complete without also discussing the period of sobriety that begins when a patient successfully ceases his or her chemical use and begins to face feelings without the benefit of a mood-altering substance. A person who stopped growing emotionally at the onset of drug abuse must face a difficult reacculturation with continued sobriety. The truth of this statement is consistently borne out by patients who become sober and begin to try to live their lives without chemical interference. Newly sober men and women in their mid-adult years respond to situations as if they were teenagers. Such patients report that they feel as if they were back in high school.

The patients who have the hardest time in sobriety are usually those who started abusing alcohol and/or drugs at an early age, come from alcoholic homes, and have a history of physical or sexual trauma. Often, these patients leave their drug of choice only to be confronted with very old and intense feelings with which they do not yet possess the skills to cope. It is this population that may do poorly in very brief detoxification stays unless additional structure and stabilization are provided to help them stay chemically free in spite of emotions they have no idea what to do with.

In well-coordinated managed care systems, the substance abuse specialist and the psychiatrist (or prescribing nurse) work closely together in the reevaluation of substance abusers once they have maintained some sobriety. Psychotropic medications are sometimes needed to help a patient address persistent depression or anxiety, or to tolerate work on issues resulting from early trauma and abuse. A team approach to care can help to keep the patient engaged with the clinician he or she has already come to trust while introducing another clinician whom the substance abuse specialist knows well.

If a patient should drop out of treatment, managed care systems are in a position to provide follow-up better then many other systems. Using the case management system, as well as communicating with the patient's medical providers (when authorized by the patient), a patient's clinician can initiate a phone conversation and encourage the patient to avoid waiting for another crisis to facilitate return to treatment. In this way, compliance can be improved and better outcomes can be achieved.

Conclusion

The links between suicidality and alcohol/drug abuse are strong. The factors accounting for this association are varied and differ from person to person. Managed care has offered us the tools for early detection of substance abuse, followed up by a coordinated range of services that could help the patient more effectively then might be possible in the traditional fee-for-service arena. For managed care to be truly responsive to this population it is essential that the elements of care mentioned in this chapter be offered. The clinician can avoid frustrating interactions with managed care preauthorization screeners by considering some of the "tips" offered in Table 6–1.

It remains important for those who treat substance abusers to recognize and anticipate the risks involved at each step of recovery and be able to involve the patient in the process of care. It is equally important that providers advocate for their patients, as for-profit health care continues to limit the care (especially the ambulatory care) and contributes to the "revolving door" syndrome we are all aware of.

Finally, as health care providers, we must be willing to accept our limitations with humility. The care of substance use disorder patients repeatedly reminds us of the boundaries of our influence and control. No matter how skillful we are or how noble our intentions may be, we may be forced at times to recognize that our task is to provide ethical health care, not to control the behavior of individuals who are competent to make their own choices.

TABLE 6–1. Clinical guidelines for working with suicidal substance abusers in a managed care setting

1. A valid assessment of suicide risk *cannot* be obtained when the patient is intoxicated.
2. Most substance abusers tend to begin to feel better once they are substance free. If they do not, the presence of comorbid psychiatric illness is more likely, increasing the risk of suicide.
3. Substance abusers in very early stages of sobriety are vulnerable to intense affect and may need additional time to learn to live with their feelings without becoming panicked. A cognitive-behavioral approach may be more helpful at first.
4. While in early recovery, substance abusers may exhibit a desire to explore their feelings before they have established the ego strength or the support network to help them cope with what they discover. Helping substance abusers slow themselves down and approach their feelings in a more thoughtful manner can be helpful.
5. Clinicians should be careful not to panic when a substance abuser, when sober, speaks of suicidal ideation. It is common for substance abusers to be frightened of their own feelings and want to stop them. If the clinician is also afraid, that increases the patient's fear and increases suicide risk.
6. Substance abusers from chaotic or dysfunctional family backgrounds may become suicidal even after 1 or 2 years of recovery. Preparing substance abusers for a range of feelings from past of present situations can help them withstand and understand intense urges to harm themselves.

TABLE 6-1. Clinical guidelines for working with suicidal substance abusers in a managed care setting *(continued)*

7. It is important for a clinician to understand the delivery system they are working with. The more familiar a clinician is with the clinical protocols and criteria for care, the better the conversation will go when negotiating with a managed system of care.
8. The clinician should establish effective working relationships with the utilization review staff who work for the managed care system. They are generally midlevel clinicians and respond to clear clinical information presented in a thoughtful manner.
9. The clincian should learn the crisis services that managed care systems use to hold and observe their patients and develop an ongoing dialogue with them. The clinician should get to know the reviewer assigned to his or her region or facility and try to develop an open-minded dialogue as more cases are reviewed.
10. The clinician should learn the limits of the managed care system he or she is working with and learn the criteria for extending benefits. The clinician should use the benefits that are available in a way that gives his or her patient the most care.

References

American Psychiatric Association: Practice guideline for the treatment of patients with substance use disorders: alcohol, cocaine, opioids. Am J Psychiatry 152 (suppl): 1–59, 1995

Brown SA, Schuckit MA: Changes in depression among abstinent alcoholics. J Stud Alcohol 49:412–417, 1988

Clark MJ, Sperry K: Suicide and cocaine. JAMA 260:2506, 1988

DeSoto CB, O'Donnell WE, DeSoto JL: Long-term recovery in alcoholics. Alcohol Clin Exp Res 13:693–697, 1989

Edmunds M, Frank R, Hogan M, et al (eds): Managing Managed Care. Washington, DC, National Academy Press, 1997

Gerstein DR, Johnson RA, Harwood HJ, et al: Evaluating recovery services: The California Drug and Alcohol Treatment Assessment (CALDATA). Fairfax, VA, Lewin VH 1 and National Opinion Research Center at the University of Chicago, 1992

Gomberg ESL: Suicide risk among women with alcohol problems. Am J Public Health 79:1363–1365, 1989

Gottschalk LA, McGuire FL, Heiser JF, et al: Suicides and homicides, in Drug Abuse Deaths in Nine Cities: A Survey Report (NIDA Research Monograph No 29). Washington, DC, U.S. Government Printing Office, 1979, pp 105–112

Helzer JE, Pryzbeck TR: The co-occurrence of alcoholism with other psychiatric disorders in the general population and its impact on treatment. J Stud Alcohol 49:219–224, 1988

Hemenway D, Solnick SJ, Colditz CA: Smoking and suicide among nurses. Am J Public Health 83:249–251, 1993

Kolozsi B: Sociology of alcoholics and their suicidal behavior in Hungary. Paper presented at the 16th annual Alcohol Epidemiology Symposium, Budapest, Hungary, June 1990

Krausz M, Degkwitz P, Haasen C, et al: Opioid addiction and suicidality. Crisis 17:175–181, 1996

McLellan AT, Aterman AI, Woody GE, et al: A quantitative measure of substance abuse treatments: the treatment services review. J Nerv Ment Dis 180:100–109, 1992

McLellan AT, Alterman A, Metzger DS, et al: Similarity of outcome predictors across opiate, cocaine, and alcohol treatments: role of treatment services. J Consult Clin Psychol 62:1141–1158, 1994

Michel K, Waeber V, Valach L, et al: A comparison of the drugs taken in fatal and nonfatal self-poisoning. Acta Psychiatr Scand 90:184–189, 1994

Miller NS, Mahler JC, Gold MS: Suicide risk associated with drug and alcohol dependence. J Addict Dis 10:49–61, 1991

Myers JK, Weissman MW, Tischler GL, et al: Six-month prevalence of psychiatric disorders in three communities. Arch Gen Psychiatry 41:959–967, 1984

National Center for Health Statistics: Vital Statistics of the United States, Vol 2, Part A: Mortality. Washington, DC, U.S. Government Printing Office, 1991, p 51 (table 1-9)

Petronis KR, Samuels JF, Moscicki EK, et al: Epidemiologic investigation of potential risk factors for suicide attempt. Soc Psychiatry Psychiatr Epidemiol 25:193–199, 1990

Schuckit MA: Genetic and clinical implications of alcoholism and affective disorder. Am J Psychiatry 143:140–147, 1986

Secretary of Health and Human Services: Seventh Special Report to the U.S. Congress on Alcohol and Health (DHHS Publ No [ADM] 90-1656). Washington, DC, U.S. Government Printing Office, 1990

Zwick WR, Bermon MD: Spectrum of services for the alcohol abusing patient, in Managed Mental Health Care. Edited by Feldman JL, Fitzpatrick RJ. Washington, DC, American Psychiatric Press, 1992, pp 273–304

CHAPTER 7

Psychiatric Pharmacotherapy, Suicide, and Managed Care

James M. Ellison, M.D., M.P.H.

The medications used to treat mental disorders have become subjects of voracious public interest. Thrusting them into public awareness, the media alternately praise their miraculous benefits and decry their terrifying dangers. In many ways, this scrutiny of pharmacotherapy serves the public well, increasing awareness of the diverse, powerful, and potentially dangerous agents newly available in our time. A less fortunate consequence of media attention has been to instill in some people an exaggerated fear that medications will precipitate insane, harmful, or self-destructive behavior. Although psychotropic medications can in most cases improve survival and facilitate recovery from mental illness, some legitimate concerns about their safety have been raised and must be appropriately acknowledged. Their rational and appropriately monitored use, moreover, is required for optimal results.

The risk of adverse outcomes to treatment, of course, is influenced by many factors. Not only the modality of treatment but also the structure and values of the system in which treatment is delivered have an impact on treatment benefits and potential risks. Managed care approaches to the treatment of mental disorders place considerable emphasis on cost-effectiveness, a value that in many systems has heavily emphasized the use of pharmacotherapy. Since pharmacotherapy lends itself logistically, if not theoretically or empirically, to delivery without psychosocial treatments and within non–mental health settings, it behooves clinicians to be aware of the risks and benefits associated with this treatment modality alone and in combination with other treatments. With few groups are pharmacotherapy treatment risks and benefits so relevant as with suicidal and parasuicidal patients.

In this chapter, I review the role of psychiatric pharmacotherapy in preventing suicide as well as the suicide risks that their use may add to treatment. I also describe aspects of managed care systems that enhance or reduce the risks of pharmacotherapy. Finally, I offer recommendations for the responsible prescribing of medications in the treatment of patients whose mental health care is insured by a managed care system.

Effects of Medications on Suicide Risk

Approximately once every 17 minutes in the United States, someone dies by suicide. In the U.S. population at large, suicide is the ninth leading cause of death, but in adolescents (see Chapter 4, this volume), the elderly (see Chapter 5), and various other subgroups, the rate of suicide is even higher. Of some reassurance in terms of preventive efforts, the highest rates occur in people with mood disorders, substance abuse disorders, and schizophrenia, many of whom are actively receiving primary care and mental health treatment.

Suicidal ideation and behavior are the end results of multiple interacting factors. They occur when an individual with particular mental vulnerabilities sustains a set of stressors that overwhelms available supports. The vulnerabilities most often include disorders from Axis I or Axis II of DSM-IV (American Psychiatric Association 1994). The mere presence of diagnoses, of course, is not sufficient to bring about suicidality, but rather the addition of stressors such as medical illness, physical pain, relationship crises, financial distress, or employment-related difficulties is often necessary to push an individual into a state of imminent danger. The pressure of these stressors must overwhelm the individual's capacity to use available supports in order for risk to reach the danger point.

Pharmacotherapy is one of the valuable supports for reducing risk, although medications sometime serve as convenient implements of self-harm and on rare occasions may even increase the risk of self-injurious behavior.

Reduction of Suicidal Ideation and Behavior With Psychiatric Pharmacotherapy

Suicidality is linked with a variety of mental disorders, especially mood disorders, schizophrenia, borderline personality disorder, and substance abuse.

Medications, used appropriately, are a powerful tool in reducing suicidality. Pharmacotherapy can intervene in psychiatric illness by counteracting or limiting a pathophysiological process, by reducing distressing suicide-promoting symptoms such as depressed or anxious mood, and by increasing coping through stabilizing mood or enhancing reality testing. Other important roles of pharmacotherapy include the reduction of physical discomfort related to side effects of concurrently prescribed medications and prophylactic use for diminishing the likelihood of relapse of a mental disorder. The role of medications in treating chronic physical pain, an important antecedent of some suicides, will not be addressed in this chapter.

There is no simple correlation between symptom reduction and reduction of suicide risk. For each of the psychiatric disorders with highest suicide risk, it appears that certain medications confer greater reduction of suicidality than others considered equally effective in treating that disorder. Lithium, for example, appears to reduce excess mortality from suicide among patients with bipolar mood disorders or schizoaffective disorder (Ahrens et al. 1995a, 1995b; Coppen et al. 1991; Nilsson 1995; Tondo et al. 1997), even when these patients are not treated in specialized lithium clinics (Nilsson 1995). Other mood regulators have not been shown to confer similar protection against suicidal behavior in mood disorder patients (Tondo et al. 1997). Indeed, lithium seems to reduce not only suicidal but also parasuicidal behavior, and this effect may be independent of satisfactory control of mood disturbance episodes (Muller-Oerlinghausen et al. 1992). Higher suicide risk appears to be linked with poor compliance (Isometsa et al. 1992). Lithium's optimal protective effect requires adequate compliance (Isometsa et al. 1992) and adequate treatment duration; in one study, for example, the substantial reduction in mortality from suicide occurred only after 2 years of continued lithium treatment (Ahrens et al. 1993). Tondo and colleagues (1997) emphasize also that cessation of lithium treatment is associated with a dramatic increase in suicidal acts, especially during the first year after discontinuation.

As many as 90% of patients with unipolar depression experience suicidal ideation (Montgomery and Åsberg 1979), and the rate of suicide attempts among depressed individuals is 80 times greater than among people with no history of psychiatric illness (Hagnell et al. 1981). Effective reduction of depressive symptoms is often, but not uniformly, associated with resolution of suicidal ideation and behavior. The serotonergic antidepressants in particular have been shown to reduce suicidal thinking. Fluvoxamine (Ottevanger 1991), paroxetine (Montgomery et al. 1995), and fluoxetine (Beasley et al. 1991; Leon et al. 1997; Muijen et al. 1988) have each been shown in controlled studies to reduce suicidal thinking and/or behavior in populations of depressed patients.

Not all treatment approaches are equally powerful in reducing suicidal ideation and behavior. Electroconvulsive therapy (ECT), for example, was shown by Avery and Winokur (1976) to reduce the risk of suicide attempts more than antidepressant treatment during the 6 months after hospital discharge. Similarly, mianserin appeared to reduce suicidal ideation more effectively than maprotiline, despite similar antidepressant efficacy, in a group of depressed patients treated under double-blind conditions (Mongtomery et al. 1978). A study that claimed greater reduction of suicidality with fluoxetine than with mianserin (Muijen et al. 1988) has been criticized on methodological grounds by Teicher and colleagues (1993).

Studies of schizophrenic and schizoaffective patients provide significant evidence that clozapine reduces suicidal ideation, plans, attempts, and completions (Meltzer and Okayli 1995; Reid et al. 1998; Walker et al. 1997). Similar effects on the suicide rate of populations of schizophrenic individuals have not been shown for other neuroleptics. Meltzer (1998) estimates that clozapine reduces suicide risk as much as 85% among schizophrenia patients and suggests that it be used even in persistently suicidal schizophrenic patients who have not shown resistance to typical neuroleptics. The reduction in mortality from suicide is so great, he argues, that clozapine's other drawbacks (e.g., adverse outcomes including agranulocytosis or toxic overdose) are outweighed. Whether the antisuicide effect of clozapine results from its lesser rate of extrapyramidal symptoms, its improvement of negative symptoms, or another action remains a matter for further investigation.

The increased rate of suicidal and parasuicidal behaviors among patients with borderline personality disorder is probably multifactorial. Trait impulsivity, comorbid depression or substance abuse (Fyer et al. 1988), anxiety disorders, adverse life circumstances, and poor support systems may all contribute. Two typical neuroleptics, flupentixol (Montgomery et al. 1992) and trifluoperazine (Cowdry and Gardner 1988), and the anticonvulsant carbamazepine (Gardner and Cowdry 1986) have been demonstrated to reduce suicidal behavior in patients with borderline personality disorder. The serotonin reuptake inhibiting antidepressants fluoxetine (Markovitz et al. 1991) and venlafaxine (Markovitz and Wagner 1995) have been shown to reduce parasuicidal self-injurious behavior among borderline patients.

As discussed in Chapter 6 of this volume, suicide risk is greatly increased among individuals with substance use disorders. The pharmacotherapy of substance abuse, however, has focused primarily on relieving comorbid disorders, supporting abstinence, or decreasing the reinforcing effects of substance abuse. Only limited data are available regarding the effects on suicidal behavior associated with pharmacotherapy of substance abuse. Such an effect might depend on reduction of concurrent mood or anxiety disorders, modulation of impulsivity or aggression, or maintenance of reality testing.

Among patients with alcohol use disorders, naltrexone has been demonstrated to be an effective therapy (Croop et al. 1997; Volpicelli et al. 1992). In addition to reducing alcohol use, it may diminish depressive symptoms in depressed alcoholic individuals (Salloum et al. 1998). How it affects risk of suicidal or parasuicidal behavior is still unknown. In contrast, disulfiram appears to be a risky agent in the treatment of suicidal alcohol abusers. As a tool for intentional self-injury, it can produce serious physical damage when combined with alcohol (Plaza Moral et al. 1986; Weissenborn et al. 1986).

Although intentional heroin overdose is rarely chosen as the means for completing a suicide, individuals who abuse opiates constitute a high-mortality group of substance abusers. Many use other substances concurrently or have comorbid depression, increasing suicide risk. In addition, accidental lethal heroin overdoses contribute another source of increased mortality in this population. Methadone maintenance has been shown to decrease the mortality rate among heroin-addicted individuals in maintenance treatment (Caplehorn et al. 1996). Although suicidality may be decreased, it is likely to remain a significant problem (Magruder-Habib et al. 1992).

Can Pharmacotherapy Increase Suicide Risk?

Pharmacotherapy does not always decrease suicidality while it alleviates symptoms of a primary mental disorder. Tranylcypromine, for example, reduced anxiety and depressive symptoms in borderline personality disorder patients without decreasing parasuicidal behavior (Cowdry and Gardner 1988). Conversely, paroxetine reduced suicidal behavior without improving mood in a group of suicidal outpatients diagnosed with various personality disorders (Verkes et al. 1998). It cannot be taken for granted that an effective pharmacotherapy of a mental disorder will also reduce the suicide risk. Indeed, there is the chilling possibility that some patients' primary mental disorders will improve at the same time as suicide risk increases. Thus, Rouillon and colleagues (1989) reported an increase in suicide rate in depressed patients treated with maprotiline, compared with those receiving placebo, despite improvement of depressive symptoms.

A further undesirable possibility, of course, is that a patient receiving pharmacotherapy will experience both a worsening of the primary disorder and an increase in suicidal behavior. Such was the finding with a subpopulation of borderline personality disorder patients who were treated with amitriptyline (Soloff et al. 1986). A different group of borderline personality disorder patients treated with alprazolam showed a large increase in self-destructive behaviors (Gardner and Cowdry 1985). Whether psychiatric medications can specifically increase the risk of suicidal behavior has been a matter of great controversy and perhaps even greater importance. If such an adverse outcome is of credible significance with particular disorders, patients, or agents, it must be considered in treatment planning and as a part of the informed consent process when treatment is offered.

Widespread public awareness that pharmacotherapy might increase suicide risk under certain circumstances developed in the wake of a report (Teicher et al. 1990) of six patients who appeared to develop suicidality after beginning fluoxetine treatment. These patients, each of whom was diagnosed with depression, were reported to develop serious suicidal ideation after 2–7 weeks of treatment with fluoxetine. Suicidality resolved within 60 to 106 days after fluoxetine was discontinued. Each patient had previously experienced suicidal ideation, though none reported such serious suicidality as during the index episode, and several denied feeling suicidal immediately prior to using fluoxetine. Two of the six patients had received fluoxetine alone, while four took one or more concurrent medications, including carbamazepine (2), neuroleptics (2), benzodiazepines (2), thyroxine (1), or stimulants (3). Each patient had previously been treated with monoamine oxidase inhibitors (MAOIs), three very recently. The patients' suicidal thoughts were described as uncharacteristic on the basis of their obsessive and violent character and an accompanying "abject acceptance and detachment" (Teicher et al. 1990). None experienced antidepressant effects.

A subsequent flurry of correspondence and case reports (Dasgupta 1990; Hoover 1990; King et al. 1991; Koizumi 1991; Masand et al. 1991; Opler 1991; Papp and Gorman 1990) brought other apparently similar cases to light. Among the many thoughtful proposed mechanisms by which fluoxetine might have facilitated treatment-emergency suicidality, the most important ones were increased risk secondary to the increase in energy associated with early antidepressant response (Feuerstein and Jackisch 1980); induction of a manic state in susceptible individuals (Brewerton 1991); "sequential pharmacodynamic interaction" by which treatment with fluoxetine would adversely affect individuals previously treated with an

MAOI (Berkley 1990); unmasking of limbic system dysfunction (Downs et al. 1991); exacerbation of OCD (Papp and Gorman 1990); induction of a serotonin syndrome (Brewerton 1991); and causation of akathisia (Chouinard 1991; Rothschild and Locke 1991; Wirshing et al. 1992). The last explanation was supported by rechallenge data from several patients (Rothschild and Locke 1991) but opposed by a large-scale study that showed no correlation of treatment-emergent suicidality with extrapyramidal adverse reactions (Tollefson et al. 1994). Other large-scale studies failed to correlate significant rates of treatment-emergent suicidality with fluoxetine treatment in populations of depressed (Beasley et al. 1991), obese (Goldstein et al. 1993), bulimic (Wheadon et al. 1992), anxiety disorder (Warshaw and Keller 1996), or obsessive-compulsive patients (Beasley et al. 1992). Though not a refutation of treatment-emergent suicidality, a large decrease in the rate of pretreatment suicidality with antidepressant treatment was confirmed by Mann and Kapur (1991). Ultimately, the American College of Neuropsychopharmacology reviewed the available data and issued a consensus statement that "a small minority of patients may experience emergent suicidal thoughts or evince such behavior during the pharmacological treatment of depression" but that "there is evidence that such emergent suicidality is not specific to any one type of antidepressant and may therefore be largely a manifestation of the natural course of the illness" ("Suicidal Behavior and Psychotropic Medication" 1993, p. 180). Concern over this issue periodically reemerges, however. For example, a recent book warns readers that treatment with serotonergic antidepressants can result in adverse neurochemical effects, including suicidal urges (Glenmullen 2000). The focus on these uncommon (if genuine) effects may, unfortunately, dissuade individuals from receiving potentially valuable treatment.

The historical importance of this controversy is that for better or worse it increased public awareness of antidepressants' potential dangers. Professional scrutiny of this issue then led to greater psychiatric awareness of earlier reports associating treatment-emergent suicidality with other antidepressants, including desipramine, nortriptyline, amoxapine, or trazodone (Damluji and Ferguson 1988) or maprotiline (Rouillon et al. 1989). Heightened attention to antidepressant effects also served to realert clinicians that other psychiatric pharmaceuticals such as diazepam (Hall and Joffe 1972) and phenobarbital (Brent et al. 1986) and nonpsychiatric pharmaceuticals such as interferon (Janssen et al. 1994) and anabolic steroids (Middleman et al. 1995) have been implicated in increasing suicide risk. In addition, a host of nonpsychiatric pharmaceuticals are known to induce or exacerbate depression, thus potentially increasing suicide risk (Bostwick 1994).

Use of Medications to Attempt or Complete Suicide

A further and very important role for pharmacotherapeutic agents among suicidal patients is their use as the implements of suicide. Indeed, among repeat suicide attempters, prescription drug overdose is the most common means chosen (Cugino et al. 1992). Benzodiazepines are a frequent choice. A Canadian study linked their use in suicide attempts to a greatly increased likelihood of past treatment for drug/alcohol abuse (Neutel and Patten 1997).

The method chosen most frequently by suicide completers, in contrast to attempters, remains firearms, while alcohol and/or benzodiazepines may serve facilitating roles. Evidence supports the assertion, initially a counterintuitive proposition, that patients who complete suicide while receiving prescribed medication are less likely to kill themselves with the medication than by some other means. A large study of suicide completers in San Diego County revealed the frequent presence of alcohol (28.3%) and benzodiazepines (33%) but a relatively low presence of antidepressants (5.9%) in the bodies of individuals who committed suicide by overdose (Mendelson and Rich 1993). Indeed, even among suicide completers known to have been treated with antidepressants, one study found that overdose with antidepressants accounted for only 14% of the suicides (Jick and Jick 1995). In 1,635 cases of suicide analyzed toxicologically among the 1,970 suicides that occurred in New York City during a 2-year study period, 17.9% of the victims died by poisoning, and the presence of antidepressants or neuroleptics was found in fewer than half of these individuals (Marzuk et al. 1995). Interestingly, nearly half of those found to have an antidepressant or neuroleptic in their bodies used lethal methods other than poisoning (Marzuk et al. 1995). The work of Isacsson and colleagues (1997) suggests that undertreatment or noncompliance contributes more to suicide risk than the effects of antidepressants. In a population of 5,281 Swedish suicide completers, many of whom were depressed, the authors found antidepressants to be detectable in only 16.5% and at toxic levels in only 4.4%. They suggested a correlation between increased antidepressant use in Sweden and an observed decrease in suicide rates.

Though benzodiazepines now emerge as a more significant overdose drug, antidepressants were rightfully regarded as the more serious poison prior to introduction of the new serotonin reuptake inhibitors (which are low in overdose toxicity; see, e.g., Phillips et al. 1997). The work of Cassidy and Henry (1987) showed that some antidepressants are more lethal than others and directed attention at desipramine—a warning consistent with the lethality ranking arrived at by Teicher and colleagues (1993). Teicher et al., using an interesting, different approach, implicated the three relatively selective noradrenergic reuptake inhibitors desipramine, nortriptyline, and maprotiline as being particularly lethal. Henry (1997) also suggested amitriptyline and dothiepin (a tricyclic antidepressant not available in the United States) to be inherently very toxic medications—a finding confirmed by Buckley and McManus (1998). In a study of interest to managed care systems that are contemplating cost from a broader perspective, D'Mello and colleagues (1995) showed that the treatment of tricyclic self-poisoning cases cost more than four times as much as the treatment of SSRI self-poisoning cases.

Many patients consult a physician shortly before attempting or completing suicide. In one study, a quarter of suicide completers consulted a doctor in the week preceding the suicide, and many were given drugs at the final consultation that were used for the purpose of overdosing (Obafunwa and Busuttil 1994). Nearly half the patients who consulted a physician in the week preceding suicide indicated suicidal intent. The rate of diagnosed psychiatric illness among this group (58.8%) was nearly 50 times greater than the rate of diagnosed psychiatric illness among the suicide completers who did not consult a physician in the week prior to suicide.

Risks of Pharmacotherapy in Managed Systems

In several different ways, managed systems encourage prescribing behaviors that could alter the risk inherent in treating suicidal patients. Managed systems affect where and by whom medications are prescribed, the dosages and quantities of medications prescribed, and what adjunctive supports are available. The implications of managed care's effects are well worth considering.

Managed systems, to a greater or lesser extent, encroach upon the specialist role of the psychiatrist with expertise in psychopharmacology in an effort to reduce costs. Primary care clinicians are encouraged to treat depression, for example, or advanced practice nurses may assume responsibility for the pharmacotherapy of patients previously referred only to a physician with advanced training in psychiatry. While this has served the valuable purpose of making treatment available to a larger population of members, some of the safeguards that previously accompanied psychiatric pharmacotherapy may now be less easily accessed.

With increasing levels of education and excellent practice guidelines to support their work, primary care clinicians can certainly prescribe antidepressants effectively for many depressed patients. At the same time, their assessment of suicide risk is likely to be less expert than that provided by an experienced mental health clinician. Primary care clinicians rarely have the time, the expertise, the therapeutic alliance, the awareness of treatment resources, or the capacity to follow up closely with a potentially suicidal patient. Many patients treated for depression in primary care settings do not have an adjunctive psychotherapist, an additional care provider who can serve as an "early warning system" for danger of self-harm. It would be of great interest to investigate whether the rate of suicide differs between similarly depressed patients treated in primary care versus specialty mental health settings.

Even a mental health specialist such as a nurse clinical specialist or psychiatrist who is prescribing in a mental health setting can find the risk of patient suicide uncomfortably altered under the current restrictions imposed by managed systems. Among the concerns raised by such specialists are these systems' emphasis on pharmacotherapy as the principal modality of treatment, sometimes unaccompanied by psychotherapy; the authorization of only brief visits and insufficiently small numbers of visits to encourage infrequent follow-ups; the imposition of formularies that may restrict clinician choices in significant ways; and the encouragement of very large (90-day or greater) prescription amounts as a means of reducing pharmacy overhead costs.

Rational Risk Management Principles and Pharmacotherapy for Suicidal Patients

Responsible prescribing within a managed care setting requires awareness of both clinical and systems issues. Clinical responsibility requires that a patient be seen with sufficient intensity to gather necessary information, assess diagnosis, plan and administer treatment, and monitor response in an adequate way. Although pharmacotherapists currently follow many different practice patterns, some patterns that have developed in some managed systems are inherently more risky for the suicidal patient's safety and expose the clinician to new levels of liability. Risk-conscious prescribers, however, can limit their exposure and maximize patient safety by following a simple set of

Psychiatric Pharmacotherapy, Suicide, and Managed Care

guidelines, summarized in Table 7–1 and discussed here with illustrative vignettes in which details have been altered for the protection of confidentiality.

TABLE 7–1. Risk-conscious pharmacotherapy for the suicidal patient in managed care

1. Base the frequency and length of pharmacotherapy appointments on the patient's needs.
2. Dispense only amounts of medications consistent with clinical needs and risks.
3. Refill prescriptions only with adequate clinical monitoring.
4. Avoid undertreatment.
5. Avoid unnecessary abrupt discontinuation of medications.
6. Choose the least toxic effective drug available.
7. Follow up on patients who miss appointments.

1. **Base the frequency and length of pharmacotherapy appointments on the patient's needs.** The professional life of a psychiatrist in many managed systems is focused on providing pharmacotherapy to a large panel of patients. Often, a group of more or less familiar psychotherapists have more frequent contact with these patients. With limited sessions authorized, the prescribing clinician's contact with the patient may be limited to as little as 15 minutes every 2–3 months—a total annual face-to-face commitment of as little as 1 hour of clinical contact. In many systems, these patients are also being managed with no or little psychotherapy (for example, 30–45 minutes every 2–4 weeks), providing very limited supportive "backup" to the "medication backup." Despite patient resistance and pressing requirements for productivity, prescribing clinicians must avoid the convenient decision to see patients less and less frequently. Visits should be scheduled often enough to allow the pharmacotherapist to monitor and document compliance with treatment, changes in mental status, and both positive and negative effects of pharmacotherapy. Clinicians who prescribe a patient's pharmacotherapy while another clinician provides psychotherapy must bear in mind that the patient's relationship with the psychotherapist does not absolve the prescribing clinician from responsibility for monitoring the patient's treatment; furthermore, the prescribing clinician should maintain ongoing communication as appropriate (and this must be with the patient's informed consent and knowledge) with the psychotherapist.

Case Example

Mr. A., a 32-year-old businessman, was evaluated by his primary care physician for depression. The primary care physician, who failed to determine that many of Mr. A.'s relatives had bipolar rather than unipolar syndromes, prescribed an antidepressant at the usual adult dosage and scheduled follow-up to take place in 1 month. The primary care physician was aware that the patient was seeing a psychotherapist but failed to contact this clinician, who could have independently alerted the primary care physician to this risky clinical scenario. By the time of the scheduled follow-up visit, Mr. A. had experienced a severely disruptive manic episode. His lack of preparedness for this complication and his lack of insight into the severity of his impaired functioning had devastating consequences when he made imprudent business and personal decisions under the influence of an adverse antidepressant response.

2. **Dispense only amounts of medication that are consistent with clinical needs and risks.** As a matter of convenience to patients and to clinicians who see them for infrequent, brief medication follow-up visits meagerly supported by infrequent psychotherapy visits with limited time for liaison between clinicians, many managed care clinicians (especially in primary care) dispense large prescriptions and/or multiple refills that will be dispensed in an unmonitored way prior to the next follow-up visit. Many mental health specialists recognize the importance of close follow-up, especially during the first weeks of pharmacotherapy for depression or anxiety disorders, but primary care clinicians' overloaded schedules may encourage use of longer follow-up intervals.

   Allowing patients to possess large numbers of potentially toxic pills is, for suicidal patients, an undesirable consequence of relying on mail-order or Internet-based pharmacy businesses that welcome 90-day prescriptions in order to reduce their own administrative costs and increase their convenience to patients. Because of the significant cost savings, patients are tempted to obtain even new medications that they have not yet found to be effective or tolerable. Sometimes only a few days or weeks of these pills are actually consumed before the trial of the medication is abandoned for various reasons, leaving the patient with a collection of unused medication that may later serve as a lethal hoard for use in overdosing. Even when the medication is at a stable maintenance dosage, the large quantities in possession at a given time present a potential hazard for an impulsive person. Improper use of these pills for excessive self-medication is often difficult to identify quickly when the patient possesses large quantities of medication.

To imperil patient safety for the sake of greater convenience is a poor choice for the clinician to make. It is better to take the time to explain to a patient the need for more careful monitoring of medication use and the decision to prescribe in smaller amounts or, on rare occasions, to entrust the medications to a third party who will dispense appropriate amounts to the patient. When compliance is in question, a patient can be asked to bring to the next appointment all pills remaining from the preceding prescription for a pill count. The validity of such a pill count depends on patient cooperation but introduces a more stringent level of monitoring.

Case Example

Mrs. B., a 65-year-old widow with failing eyesight and impaired mobility, requested her nurse clinical specialist to prescribe 90 days of the new antidepressant she was going to start. The nurse understood that this would be more convenient and affordable and that going to the pharmacy was difficult, but chose instead to dispense a 2-week medication sample. If the medication was well tolerated, the patient could follow up by telephone and the HMO pharmacy would mail a larger prescription to her home.

3. **Refill prescriptions only with adequate clinical monitoring.** Some patients attempt to limit their copayment expenses and to save time by missing scheduled appointments and then telephoning for a refill. Others may be too disorganized to comply with appointments. In either scenario, this is a high-risk situation for both patient and prescriber, because medications should not be routinely refilled without adequate monitoring. A crucial component of adequate medical monitoring is for the clinician to be aware of changes in the patient's medical health or use of concurrent drugs or prescribed medications that may alter the effects or safety of the psychiatric pharmacotherapy.

    Some patients visit their primary care physician or psychiatrist with the specific goal of obtaining lethal medication for the purpose of overdosing. A study of Finnish cases of suicide found that neuroleptics and antidepressants used for suicide were, in the majority of cases, the victims' own prescribed drugs (Ohlberg et al. 1996). Among a group of patients with medical contact during the week before suicide, 43% requested a prescription refill, and three-quarters of these simply collected a refill prescription and did not speak with a doctor (Obafunwa and Busuttil 1994).

Case Example

Mr. C. hated interrupting his busy work schedule to visit the psychiatrist for a prescription refill. After many heated discussions, the psychiatrist was tempted simply to write a large prescription and schedule semi-annual visits as the patient requested. Awareness of this individual's instability, however, led the psychiatrist instead to initiate a collaborative relationship with a second clinician who was able to provide psychotherapy in evening appointments that were more acceptable to the patient. In between the bimonthly medication appointments, the patient kept in touch with the psychiatrist by telephone or e-mail, and the psychiatrist was in touch with the psychotherapist as appropriate.

4. **Avoid undertreatment.** Despite public concern about overuse of medications, it is still more typical to see patients with depression, anxiety, or psychosis undertreated rather than overtreated. Subtherapeutic levels of medication create the illusion that effective care is being provided, preventing actual appropriate treatment from being delivered. Attention to compliance and familiarity with usual therapeutic dose ranges are necessary for optimal prescribing. When a nonresponder to treatment appears to be treatment-compliant, plasma drug level measurements can increase the likelihood that adequate levels of medication will be prescribed.

Case Example

Ms. D. was seen only every 3 months by the primary care physician who prescribed a benzodiazepine for her panic disorder with agoraphobia. After several years of this infrequent treatment, her family pressured her into attending psychotherapy sessions and her psychotherapist obtained permission to contact the primary care physician. The psychotherapist helped the primary care physician understand that the patient's lack of complaints or requests between sessions arose from her withdrawn and limited functional level rather than from a successful treatment. Her pharmacotherapy was transferred to the anxiety disorders specialty clinic of the MCO (managed care organization), where she was seen more frequently for the interim while her medication was changed and the dosage was adjusted, in collaboration with her psychotherapist's input.

5. **Avoid unnecessary abrupt discontinuation of medications.** Many pharmacotherapeutic agents, but particularly the anticholinergic tricyclics (Dilsaver 1989), the short-acting serotonin reuptake inhibitors (Zajecka et al. 1997), and the shorter-acting benzodiazepines, are associated with unpleasant discontinuation syndromes. The abrupt cessa-

tion of sedative-hypnotics can also be quite dangerous, even life-threatening. Adequate access to a prescribing clinician is required in order to avert this avoidable complication of treatment.

Case Example

When Mr. E. missed his appointment, he called to reschedule and was told by the clinic receptionist that nothing was available for the next month. He had three more weeks of pills (a short-acting serotonin reuptake inhibitor that he took as a treatment for his depression) and did not want to be perceived as demanding, so he quietly accepted this apparently routine rescheduling and did not ask for a refill. By the time he was seen, he was experiencing severe nausea and dizziness. He wished he had known how uncomfortable this withdrawal would be, and he was very reluctant to resume the medication that he considered to have caused this intense physical distress.

6. **Choose the least toxic effective drug available.** Use of formularies and mandatory interchange policies have become routine in managed care oriented pharmacies. The result can be encouragement of the clinician to prescribe a drug that is cheaper on a unit-cost basis but possessed of a distinctly more toxic side-effect profile. Until recently, for example, some managed care plans required clinicians to obtain preauthorization to treat a depressed patient with a newer serotonergic antidepressant instead of a tricyclic agent. Currently, some plans encourage their empaneled clinicians to prescribe higher-dosage forms (e.g., sertraline 100-mg tablet rather than 25- or 50-mg tablets) that can be broken by the patient into smaller doses. An additional constraint faces patients on Medicaid whose prescriptions are not reimbursed.

   The choice of which medication to use and which dosage tablet to prescribe should take into account clinical issues. The manufacturing companies provide in various ways for the assistance of patients who lack the means to purchase their medications. When more toxic drugs such as tricyclic antidepressants or MAOIs are used, appropriate patient education must be provided and patient prescreening and precautions should be taken.

Case Example

Ms. F.'s managed insurance relied on a formulary that included two serotonin reuptake inhibitors, one of which had elicited in her an unpleasant tachycardic reaction. Because the copayment for a prescription of a newer alternative antidepressant would be larger than for the other serotonin reuptake inhibitor, the prescribing psychiatrist chose to "take a chance" with a low dose of the second serotonin reuptake inhibitor. Sure enough, a tachycardic anxious reaction developed even at the low dose. Subsequent treatment with the newer alternative medication was a little more expensive but far more effective.

7. **Follow up on patients who miss appointments.** In systems that serve a high volume of patients with infrequent visits, systems are often (and always should be!) developed for identifying patients who fail to show for a scheduled appointment. More difficult to monitor are those patients who cancel an approaching pharmacotherapy appointment but fail to reschedule. The anonymity of some large health care systems allows these patients to vanish from follow-up until a crisis or relapse forces their needs again into clinical awareness. This is especially problematic in managed systems that divide therapy, assigning pharmacotherapy to one clinician and psychotherapy to another, or with patients who receive only pharmacotherapy. It is valuable to institute a system that alerts pharmacotherapists both to patients who miss appointments and to those who do not reschedule.

Case Example

Mr. G., an elderly widower, considerately called ahead to cancel his appointment with the primary care physician who prescribed medication for his depression. He was feeling too weak to attend the appointment and offered to call back when stronger. Although he dropped off the list of scheduled appointments, his weakness (which was a manifestation of his depression) continued to increase. By the time that Mr. G. had taken to bed for such an extended period, the accumulating mail in his box led a thoughtful neighbor to intervene in time to avert a potentially lethal outcome. As a result of this experience, the MCO's mental health clinic devised a system for notifying clinicians when patients had "dropped off the schedule" due to cancellation of an appointment without rescheduling.

Conclusion

The growing refinement of pharmacotherapy and its increasing provision under managed care systems have been linked with the delivery of pharmacotherapy by primary care clinicians less attuned to psychiatric treatment issues; with specialist visits that are briefer, less integrated with a comprehensive treatment plan, and spaced further apart; and with prescribing habits that place greater responsibility on patients to safeguard their medications and use them appropriately. Under these conditions, it is necessary for prescribers to consider the risks associated with the treatment and to adopt safety-conscious, risk-conscious practices in their prescribing.

References

Ahrens B, Muller-Oerlinghausen B, Grof P: Length of lithium treatment needed to eliminate the high mortality of affective disorders. Br J Psychiatry 21(suppl):27–29, 1993

Ahrens B, Grof P, Moller HJ, et al: Extended survival of patients on long-term lithium treatment. Can J Psychiatry 40:241–246, 1995a

Ahrens B, Muller-Oerlinghausen B, Schou M, et al: Excess cardiovascular and suicide mortality of affective disorders may be reduced by lithium prophylaxis. J Affect Disord 33:67–75, 1995b

American Psychiatric Association: Diagnostic and Statistical Manual of Mental Disorders, 4th Edition. Washington, DC, American Psychiatric Association, 1994

Avery D, Winokur G: Mortality in depressed patients treated with electroconvulsive and antidepressants. Arch Gen Psychiatry 33:1029–1337, 1976

Beasley CM Jr, Dornseif BE, Bosomworth JC, et al: Fluoxetine and suicide: a meta-analysis of controlled trials of treatment for depression. BMJ 303:685–692, 1991

Beasley CM Jr, Potvin JH, Masica DN, et al: Fluoxetine: no association with suicidality in obsessive-compulsive disorder. J Affect Disord 24:1–10, 1992

Berkley RB: Discussion of fluoxetine and suicidal tendencies (letter). Am J Psychiatry 147:1572, 1990

Bostwick JM: Neuropsychiatry of depression, in The Psychotherapist's Guide to Neuropsychiatry. Edited by Ellison JM, Weinstein CS, Hodel-Malinofsky T. Washington, DC, American Psychiatric Press, 1994, pp 409–431

Brent DA: Overrepresentation of epileptics in a consecutive series of suicide attempters seen at a children's hospital, 1978–1983. Journal of the American Academy of Child Psychiatry 25:242–246, 1986

Brewerton TD: Fluoxetine-induced suicidality, serotonin, and seasonality. Biol Psychiatry 30:190–196, 1991

Buckley NA, McManus PR: Can the fatal toxicity of antidepressant drugs be predicted with pharmacological and toxicological data? Drug Saf 18:369–381, 1998

Caplehorn JR, Dalton MS, Haldar F, et al: Methadone maintenance and addicts' risk of fatal heroin overdose. Subst Use Misuse 31:177–196, 1996

Cassidy S, Henry J: Fatal toxicity of antidepressant drugs in overdose. Br Med J 295:1021–1024, 1987

Chouinard G: Fluoxetine and preoccupation with suicide (letter). Am J Psychiatry 148:1258–1259, 1991

Coppen A, Standish-Barry H, Bailey J, et al: Does lithium reduce the mortality of recurrent mood disorders? J Affect Disord 23:1–7, 1991

Cowdry RW, Gardner DL: Pharmacotherapy of borderline personality disorder: alprazolam, carbamazepine, trifluoperazine, and tranylcypromine. Arch Gen Psychiatry 45:111–119, 1988

Croop RS, Faulkner EB, Labriola DF: The safety profile of naltrexone in the treatment of alcoholism: results from a multicenter usage study. The Naltrexone Usage Study Group. Arch Gen Psychiatry 54:1130–1135, 1997

Cugino A, Markovich EI, Rosenblatt S, et al: Searching for a pattern: repeat suicide attempts. J Psychosoc Nurs Ment Health Serv 30:23–26, 1992

D'Mello DA, Finkbeiner DS, Kocher KN: The cost of antidepressant overdose. Gen Hosp Psychiatry 17:454–455, 1995

Damluji NF, Ferguson JM: Paradoxical worsening of depressive symptomatology caused by antidepressants. J Clin Psychopharmacol 8:347–349, 1988

Dasgupta K: Additional cases of suicidal ideation associated with fluoxetine. Am J Psychiatry 147:1570, 1990

Dilsaver SC: Antidepressant withdrawal syndromes: phenomenology and pathophysiology. Acta Psychiatr Scand 79:113–117, 1989

Downs J, Ward J, Farmer R: Preoccupation with suicide in patients treated with fluoxetine (letter; comment). Am J Psychiatry 148:1090–1091, 1991

Feuerstein TJ, Jackisch R: Why do some antidepressants promote suicide? (letter). Psychopharmacology (Berl) 90:422, 1980

Fyer MR, Frances AJ, Sullivan T, et al: Suicide attempts in patients with borderline personality disorder. Am J Psychiatry 145:737–739, 1988

Gardner DL, Cowdry RW: Alprazolam-induced dyscontrol in borderline personality disorder. Am J Psychiatry 142:98–100, 1985

Gardner DL, Cowdry RW: Positive effects of carbamazepine on behavioral dyscontrol in borderline personality disorder. Am J Psychiatry 143:519–522, 1986

Glenmullen J: Prozac Backlash: Overcoming the Dangers of Prozac, Zoloft, Paxil, and Other Antidepressants With Safe, Effective Alternatives. New York, Simon & Schuster, 2000

Goldstein DJ, Rampey AH, Potvin JH, et al: Analyses of suicidality in double-blind, placebo-controlled trials of pharmacotherapy for weight reduction. J Clin Psychiatry 54:309–316, 1993

Hagnell O, Lanke J, Rorsman B: Suicide rates in the Lundby study. Mental illness as a risk factor for suicide. Neuropsychobiology 7:248–253, 1981

Hall RC, Joffe JR: Aberrant response to diazepam: a new syndrome. Am J Psychiatry 129:738–742, 1972

Henry JA: Epidemiology and relative toxicity of antidepressant drugs in overdose. Drug Saf 16:374–390, 1997

Hoover CE: Additional cases of suicidal ideation associated with fluoxetine (letter; comment). Am J Psychiatry 147:1570–1571, 1990

Isacsson G, Holmgren P, Druid H, et al: The utilization of antidepressant—a key issue in the prevention of suicide: an analysis of 5281 suicides in Sweden during the period 1992–1994. Acta Psychiatr Scand 96:94–100, 1997

Isometsa E, Henriksson M, Lonnqvist J: Completed suicide and recent lithium treatment. J Affect Disord 26:101–103, 1992

Janssen HL, Brouwer JT, van der Mast RC, et al: Suicide associated with alpha-interferon therapy for chronic viral hepatitis. J Hepatol 21:241–243, 1994

Jick SS, Dean AD, Jick H: Antidepressants and suicide. BMJ 310:215–218, 1995

King RA, Riddle MA, Chappell PB, et al: Emergence of self-destructive phenomena in children and adolescents during fluoxetine treatment. J Am Acad Child Adolesc Psychiatry 30:179–186, 1991

Koizumi H: Fluoxetine and suicidal ideation (letter). J Am Acad Child Adolesc Psychiatry 30:695, 1991

Leon AC, Keller MB, Warshaw MG, et al: A prospective study of fluoxetine treatment and suicidal behavior in affectively-ill subjects. Am J Psychiatry 156:195–201, 1997

Magruder-Habib K, Hubbard RL, Ginzburg HM: Effects of drug misuse treatment on symptoms of depression and suicide. Int J Addict 27:1035–1065, 1992

Mann JJ, Kapur S: The emergence of suicidal ideation and behavior during antidepressant pharmacotherapy. Arch Gen Psychiatry 48:1027–1033, 1991

Markovitz PJ, Wagner SC: Venlafaxine in the treatment of borderline personality disorder. Psychopharmacol Bull 31:773–777, 1995

Markovitz PJ, Calabrese JR, Schulz SC, et al: Fluoxetine in the treatment of borderline and schizotypal personality disorders. Am J Psychiatry 148:1064–1067, 1991

Marzuk PM, Tardiff K, Leon AC, et al: Use of prescription psychotropic drugs among suicide victims in New York City. Am J Psychiatry 152:1520–1522, 1995

Masand P, Gupta S, Dewan M: Suicidal ideation related to fluoxetine treatment (letter). N Engl J Med 324:420, 1991

Meltzer HY: Suicide in schizophrenia: risk factors and clozapine treatment. J Clin Psychiatry 59 (no 3, suppl):15–20, 1998

Meltzer HY, Okayli G: Reduction of suicidality during clozapine treatment of neuroleptic-resistant schizophrenia: impact on risk-benefit assessment. Am J Psychiatry 151:1744–1752, 1995

Mendelson WB, Rich CL: Sedatives and suicide: The San Diego Study. Acta Psychiatr Scand 88:337–41, 1993

Middleman AB, Faulkner AH, Woods ER, et al: High-risk behaviors among high school students in Massachusetts who use anabolic steroids. Pediatrics 96:268–272, 1995

Montgomery SA, Åsberg M: A new depression rating scale designed to be sensitive to change. Br J Psychiatry 134:382–389, 1979

Montgomery SA, Crohnolm B, Åsberg M, et al: Differential effects on suicidal ideation of mianserin, maprotiline and amitriptyline. Br J Clin Pharmacol 5 (suppl 1):77S–80S, 1978

Montgomery SA, Montgomery DB, Green M, et al: Pharmacotherapy in the prevention of suicidal behavior. J Clin Psychopharmacol 12 (no 2, suppl):27S–31S, 1992

Montgomery SA, Dunner DL, Dunbar GC: Reduction of suicidal thoughts with paroxetine in comparison with reference antidepressants and placebo. Eur Neuropsychopharmacol 5:5–13, 1995

Muijen M, Silverstone T, Mehmet A, et al: A comparative clinical trial of fluoxetine, mianserin, and placebo in depressed outpatients. Acta Psychiatr Scand 78:384–390, 1988

Muller-Oerlinghausen B, Muser-Causemann B, Volk J: Suicides and parasuicides in a high-risk patient group on and off lithium long-term medication. J Affect Disord 25:261–269, 1992

Neutel CI, Patten SB: Risk of suicide attempts after benzodiazepine and/or antidepressant use. Ann Epidemiol 7:568–574, 1997

Nilsson A: Mortality in recurrent mood disorders during periods on and off lithium. A complete population study in 362 patients. Pharmacopsychiatry 28:8–13, 1995

Obafunwa JO, Busuttil A: Clinical contract preceding suicide. Postgrad Med J 70:428–432, 1994

Ohlberg A, Vuori E, Ojanpera I, et al: Alcohol and drugs in suicides. Br J Psychiatry 169:75–80, 1996

Opler LA: Fluoxetine and preoccupation with suicide (letter). Am J Psychiatry 148:1259, 1991

Ottevanger EA: Fluvoxamine activity profile with special emphasis on the effect on suicidal ideation. Eur J Clin Res 1:47–54, 1991

Papp LA, Gorman JM: Suicidal preoccupation during fluoxetine treatment (letter; comment). Am J Psychiatry 147:1380–1381, 1990

Phillips S, Brent J, Kulig K, et al: Fluoxetine versus tricyclic antidepressants: a prospective multicenter study of antidepressant drug overdoses. The Antidepressant Study Group. J Emerg Med 15:439–445, 1997

Plaza Moral V, Fernandez Sola J, Nogue Xarau S: [Acute myocardial infarction and diffuse cerebral ischemia after attempted suicide with ethanol and disulfiram]. Rev Clin Esp 179:223–224, 1986 [in Spanish]

Reid WH, Mason M, Hogan T: Suicide prevention effects associated with clozapine therapy in schizophrenia and schizoaffective disorder. Psychiatr Serv 49:1029–1033, 1998

Rosenbaum JF, Fava M: Suicidality and fluoxetine: is there a relationship? J Clin Psychiatry 52:108–111, 1991

Rothschild AJ, Locke CA: Reexposure to fluoxetine after serious suicide attempts by three patients: the role of akathisia. J Clin Psychiatry 52:491–493, 1991

Rouillon F, Phillips R, Serrurier D, et al: Rechutes de depression unipolaire et efficacite de al maprotiline. L'Encephale 15:527–534, 1989

Salloum IM, Cornelius JR, Thase ME, et al: Naltrexone utility in depressed alcoholics. Psychopharmacol Bull 34:111–115, 1998

Soloff PH, George A, Nathan RS, et al: Paradoxical effects of amitriptyline on borderline patients. Am J Psychiatry 143:1603–1605, 1986

Suicidal behavior and psychotropic medication. Accepted as a consensus statement by the ACNP Council, March 2, 1992. Neuropsychopharmacology 8:177–183, 1993

Teicher MH, Glod C, Cole JO: Emergence of intense suicidal preoccupation during fluoxetine treatment. Am J Psychiatry 147:207–210, 1990

Teicher MH, Glod CA, Cole JO: Antidepressants and the emergence of suicidal tendencies. Drug Saf 8:186–212, 1993

Tollefson GD, Rampey AH, Beasley CM Jr, et al: Absence of a relationship between adverse events and suicidality during pharmacotherapy for depression. J Clin Psychopharmacol 14:163–169, 1994

Tondo L, Jamison KR, Baldessarini RJ: Effect of lithium maintenance on suicidal behavior in major mood disorders. Ann N Y Acad Sci 826:339–351, 1997

Verkes RJ, Van der Mast RC, Hengeveld MW, et al: Reduction by paroxetine of suicidal behavior in patients with repeated suicide attempts but not major depression. Am J Psychiatry 155:543–547, 1998

Volpicelli JR, Alterman AI, Hayashida M, et al: Naltrexone in the treatment of alcohol dependence. Arch Gen Psychiatry 49:876–880, 1992

Walker AM, Lanza LL, Arellano A, et al: Mortality in current and former users of clozapine. Epidemiology 8:671–677, 1997

Warshaw MG, Keller MB: The relationship between fluoxetine use and suicidal behavior in 654 subjects with anxiety disorders. J Clin Psychiatry 57:158–166, 1996

Weissenborn K, Peters J, Heinze HJ et al: [Brain infarct and polyradiculitis as a sequela of attempted suicide with disulfiram. Nervenarzt 57:159–162, 1986 [in German]

Wheadon DE, Rampey AH Jr, Thompson VL, et al: Lack of association between fluoxetine and suicidality in bulimia nervosa. J Clin Psychiatry 53:235–241, 1992

Wirshing WC, Van Putten T, Rosenberg J, et al: Fluoxetine, akathisia, and suicidality: is there a causal connection? (letter). Arch Gen Psychiatry 49:580–581, 1992

Zajecka J, Tracy KA, Mitchell S: Discontinuation symptoms after treatment with serotonin reuptake inhibitors: a literature review. J Clin Psychiatry 58:291–297, 1997

CHAPTER 8

Risk Management Issues for Clinicians Who Treat Suicidal Patients in Managed Systems

Catherine Keyes, J.D.

Risk is inherent in the treatment of suicidal patients, and the legal risks faced by mental health clinicians who treat suicidal patients can be magnified by the requirements of managed care. Areas of risk can be defined and summarized, minimized by good practices, even insured against, but unfortunately never entirely eliminated. Optimal clinical risk management, therefore, depends on the delivery of compassionate care that incorporates current standards of practice and relevant advances in professional knowledge and technology rather than defensive measures aimed at limiting exposure to liability. In this chapter, therefore, I identify areas of risk and suggest risk management strategies while acknowledging the impossibility of eliminating risk from work with suicidal patients.

Many of the principles discussed in this chapter will be illustrated by referring to case law (i.e., findings arising from specific legal proceedings). The standards governing liability, however, are less uniform than this method of discussion might suggest. Conclusions drawn from one case or in one jurisdiction may not be upheld in apparently similar circumstances elsewhere.

Negligence and Standard of Care

The concept of *negligence* embodies the way in which the legal system holds people accountable for the harm their actions cause when they are less careful than society expects them to be. The victim of another's negligence can seek compensation, usually in the form of money, as a way of becoming "whole" again. For the potentially negligent, by contrast, the threat of having to pay money is intended to deter irresponsible behavior.

How careful does society expect us to be? The lawyerly answer to this question is: In general, a person is expected to be *reasonably* careful. Physicians are members of a profession that demands and fosters a high level of trust from clients (Zaremski and Goldstein 1988–1990, Vol. 1, §6:03), and therefore they are held to a standard that reflects the magnitude of this trust.

The duty of care expected of other mental health professionals depends on the degree of skill and care associated with their professional credentials and roles. For each discipline, there is a discipline-specific level of reasonable care. Psychiatrists, for example, have a duty to treat their patients with the skill, diligence, and due care that a qualified psychiatrist would provide when acting under the same or similar circumstances, while psychologists are held to the levels of skill and care of qualified psychologists (Packman and Harris 1998).

In certain cases, care that reflects current practice may not be sufficient to protect against liability. This was articulated, for example, in *Helling v. Carey* (1974), a landmark case that attributed negligence to an ophthalmologist for failing to administer a glaucoma "puff test" to a 32-year-old woman who subsequently lost her vision. Despite substantial testimony that ophthalmologists did not routinely give this test to patients of her age, the court held that a professional should not be shielded from liability just because his whole profession lags behind in the use of an available technology. In the context of caring for suicidal patients in managed systems, such a ruling suggests that managed care clinicians who curtail medically necessary treatment solely because such denial is common practice may not be shielded from liability by the similar behavior of their peers.

Though many supervisors may not realize this, trainees in each discipline are held to the standard of the fully trained in order to protect the welfare of patients. Mental health trainees, therefore, are expected to conform to the standard of care of *professionals* who are competent to practice in their specialty (Helms and Helms 1991). Psychiatric interns or residents, for example, are held to the standard appropriate for fully licensed psychiatrists. Nurses in training for advanced practice certification are held to the standard of care and skill of certified advanced practice nurses.[1] Clinicians responsible for assessing trainees' skills and monitoring the care they provide may be unaware of the considerable responsibility this standard places on the supervisor.

Whether by action or inaction, the harm that comes to a patient as a direct result of the clinician's violation of the duty to provide reasonable care is considered *malpractice* (Simon 1992). Malpractice and negligence, terms often used as though interchangeable, are not truly synonymous. A patient can sue a mental health professional for malpractice, for example, under theories other than negligence, including slander, breach of contract, or battery. Furthermore, malpractice insurance may not cover all aspects of professional negligence: mental health care professional liability insurers often exclude coverage for boundary violations, whether they are intentional or the result of inadvertently negligent management of transference/countertransferrence issues.

Gutheil (1998, p. 252) suggests that failure to provide appropriate care often does not result in a malpractice lawsuit; rather, malpractice lawsuits typically arise from a "malignant synergy" of bad outcomes and bad feelings. This theory would explain, in part, the small overlap between cases in which actual harm has been caused by clinician negligence and cases in which a malpractice lawsuit has been filed. The Harvard Medical Practice Study confirmed this discrepancy, finding that many instances of clinician negligence do not lead to malpractice suits, while many malpractice suits do not reveal evidence of negligence (Brennan et al. 1991).

Few outcomes compare with suicide attempts or completed suicide in their capacity to create bad feelings, suggesting an explanation for the high incidence of suicide-related malpractice suits against mental health providers. ProMutual Group (1997), a Massachusetts-based malpractice insurer, analyzed 188 claims alleging psychiatrists' negligence between 1987 and 1996. It found that the most frequent allegation, raised in 25% of the cases, was failure to prevent suicide and/or homicide. A similar study by CNA HealthPro of approximately 200 of its behavioral health care claims closed between 1990 and 1996 found the allegation of *failure to monitor resulting in suicide* in 16% of approximately 200 of its behavioral health care claims closed between 1990 and 1996 (Brytan and Davis 1997). This rate was exceeded only by the allegation of failure to diagnose/making the wrong diag-

---

[1] See, for example, *Central Anesthesia Associates, P.C. v. Worthy*, a 1985 case rejecting the argument that a student nurse anesthetist should be held only to the standard of care and skill of a second-year student nurse anesthetist.

nosis, which was present in 35% of cases (Brytan and Davis 1997).

However bad the feelings and outcome, though, a plaintiff who alleges negligence cannot prevail in court without proving that

- The clinician owed him or her a duty;
- The clinician breached the standard of care;
- The plaintiff was harmed; and
- The harm was a foreseeable result of the breach.

Cases that allege negligence in the treatment of suicidal patients most often turn on the question of whether the defendant breached the duty to provide care that met the appropriate standard. In order to determine whether there has indeed been a breach of duty, there must be some agreement about what that duty entails. Because circumstances vary and patients' situations differ, the standard of care is articulated in a general way. When questions arise in specific malpractice suits, the standard is clarified by means of expert testimony from individuals in the same field as the clinician defendant. An overview (Annotation *American Law Reports* 1997) of mental health malpractice liability described the standard of care for "one assuming to diagnose and treat mental illness" as "generally that of ordinary professional skill and care as employed in the locality, bearing in mind the patient's known condition and the advanced state of the profession at the time of treatment" (p. 604). In a 1998 malpractice case (*Sheeley v. Memorial Hospital* 1998), the Rhode Island Supreme Court noted a trend away from this "locality rule" and joined the majority of states in holding physicians to a national, rather than local, standard of care. I will therefore discuss the nature of the clinician's duty in some detail, giving examples of specific areas of duty and providing additional, briefer comments on harm and foreseeability. I will also consider implications for clinicians in managed systems.

The Clinician's Duty

Duty, or the requirement to act as a prudent professional, arises whenever the clinician interacts with a patient. Some clinicians unwittingly enter into these relationships, perhaps by giving medical advice to fellow guests at a cocktail party or by writing prescriptions for friends who want to avoid health insurance hassles or the delay until an appointment can be made. Among mental health care providers, there is the widespread misperception that a provider/patient relationship is not created unless or until the patient

Risk Management Issues

pays a fee. In fact, although a fee may assist in establishing appropriate provider/patient boundaries, the absence of a fee does not rule out the existence of a provider/patient relationship and duty.

With respect to the suicidal patient, several important aspects of duty typically bear on whether the standard of care has been met by the clinician.

Duty to Protect

Psychiatrists and psychiatric hospitals have a "special relationship" to hospitalized patients, a relationship that imposes a duty to protect them against foreseeable harm, including suicide (Wilkinson 1998). Mental health care professionals are not and cannot be guarantors of their patients' safety, even in the hospital setting, but they have been found liable for failing to take adequate precautions (Packman and Harris 1998). Thus, a psychiatrist was not liable when, while passing through and closing a locked ward door, a suicidal patient bolted from a room 15 feet away, ran past him, then jumped out a nearby window (*Gregory v. Robinson* 1960). The court considered the psychiatrist's precautions adequate, including his brief but thorough glance around the ward to ascertain the position of the patient, and his attempt to hasten through the automatic door during which he looked away from the patient for only 1 or 2 seconds. On the other hand, hospital staff were found liable when a suicidal patient jumped from the roof of a parking garage while out of the hospital on a pass (*Huntley v. State* 1984). In that case, the patient discussed her suicide plan in detail with a hospital staff member 1 day before she was granted off-premises privileges, but the staff member did not relay the information to the staff psychiatrist.

This special relationship has been found in the outpatient setting as well, although courts acknowledge that mental health professionals have limited ability to exercise control over patients who are not eligible for involuntary commitment (*Bellah v. Greenson* 1978; *Farwell v. Un* 1990; "Liability for Patient Suicide" 1994).[2]

Duty to Exercise Proper Judgment in Making Diagnosis and Treatment Decisions

Mental health care professionals are expected to exercise proper judgment in making diagnosis and treatment decisions. Fundamental to this process is the need to gather and evaluate information about the patient's mental sta-

---

[2]For a state-by-state analysis of cases in which it is alleged that a psychiatrist or psychologist failed to take appropriate steps to prevent a patient's suicide, see Annotation *American Law Reports* 1998 and 1991 supplement.

tus. The case of *Bell v. New York City Health & Hospitals Corp.* (1982), in which a patient doused himself in gasoline and set himself on fire after he was released from involuntary hospitalization, is illustrative because the psychiatrist was found to have inadequately assessed the patient's mental status prior to discharging him. The court in *Bell* faulted the psychiatrist for not trying to procure the patient's previous treatment records despite the patient's refusal to discuss his psychiatric history. The records, it was later shown, revealed three prior suicide attempts. The court found troubling the psychiatrist's failure to investigate the patient's hallucinations, delusions, and preoccupation with Jesus Christ—a lapse that may have been explained but not excused by his failure to read the notes entered in the medical record by the nursing staff. Describing the relationship between assessment and professional judgment, the court stated that

> [p]hysicians are not liable for mistakes in professional judgment, provided that they do what they think best *after careful examination*. . . . However, liability can ensue if their judgment *is not based upon intelligence* and thus there is a failure to exercise any professional judgment. [emphasis in original]

Another New York case elucidates the elements of adequate assessment, even as it acknowledges the possibility for error. In *Timmins v. State* (1968), a psychiatric patient was allowed to leave the hospital for home visits when accompanied by either his wife or his brother. During one of these visits, the patient killed his 3-year-old daughter. A lawsuit followed, and the court found the psychiatrists properly obtained the patient's history, treated and tested the patient, observed improvement in his condition, and contemplated the therapeutic value of granting him off-site privileges. The psychiatrists' decision was an honest error of professional judgment, but not the basis for liability (Wilkinson 1998).

The medical record plays a remarkably important role in cases pertaining to the assessment and care of suicidal patients. The *Bell* court's dissatisfaction with the provider's failure to review previous or contemporaneous treatment records is echoed in the case of *Cohen v. State of New York* (1976). This case involved an attending psychiatrist who discussed a suicidal patient's progress with her supervisee, a first-year resident, and with other staff members before recommending the patient be discharged, but kept little record of these interactions. The court found that "there is nothing in the hospital records to support a finding that she ever made a medical judgment fully based upon the nurses' notes and any kind of personal interview." This observation reflects not simply an expectation that a provider will read a patient's record as part of the assessment process, but an understanding that, in the inpatient setting at least, the record is the means of communication among providers and requires appropriate entries by the various team members. The duty to document is also highlighted in the case of *Abille v. United States* (1980), in which a hospitalized, suicidal patient was treated as if his status had improved and was granted privileges reflecting the assumed change. While traveling unescorted to breakfast, the patient entered an unguarded building and jumped out of a seventh-floor window. The psychiatrist and the nurses believed the psychiatrist had evaluated the patient and ordered the change in status, but there was no record of the order, although one would have been required by hospital policy. In fact, both the plaintiff's and defendant's expert in this case agreed that the psychiatrist's failure to "keep contemporary progress notes reflecting his exercise of judgment, and the basis for it, was below the standard of care." Liability for the patient's suicide was attributed to the defendant psychiatrist on this basis alone— a warning to those who document poorly or not at all.

Mental health professionals occasionally justify maintaining few records or making only terse notations as a means of protecting patients' confidentiality, but this practice carries its own risks. In *Brandvain v. Ridgeview Institute, Inc.* (1988, aff'd 1989), the mental health providers, perhaps guarding the confidentiality of a second-year resident who admitted himself to a hospital for substance abuse treatment, left his record detrimentally bare. The admitting physician in *Brandvain* did not note in the record the patient's recent suicide attempt as described to him by the patient's wife. None of the many providers who knew about the patient's attempt to hang himself on the fourth day of his hospitalization documented the incident or the basis for concluding that this action was a gesture not warranting suicide precautions. Staff put the patient on 15-minute checks, which they communicated by word of mouth to the next shift but did not mention in the medical record. Two shifts later, the word-of-mouth system fell apart, the nurse did not perform the 15-minute checks, and the patient hanged himself from a shower handgrip. The medical record did not confirm the level of care that the staff intended to provide.

Although managed health care systems may create stressful time pressures for mental health care professionals, such conditions do not alter the duty to gather information necessary for appropriate decision making. Accessing treatment records, integrating information from a variety of sources, and effectively communicating salient information to team members may, in fact, be more important in this context than in the fee-for-service environment. After all, the most basic expectation of patients is that their care will be *managed* in the sense of an adequate gathering of information, a diagnostic decision, a treatment planning process, and implementation of the treatment plan. Failure to *manage* the care in this sense could easily precipitate the bad feelings that combine so poorly with bad outcomes.

Lessons learned from cases involving assessment of suicidal patients suggest the following risk management strategies:

- With the patient's permission, request prior treatment records.
- If prior treatment records become available and you have permission, review them.
- If either inpatient or outpatient mental health care is provided by a team, require the team members to make contemporaneous notes and to read the notes made by others.
- Documentation augments but does not replace oral communication. Identify serious concerns by speaking with appropriate other team members as well as by communicating in notes.
- Document comments and concerns expressed by family members and significant others that elucidate the patient's mental state.
- Document relevant suicide risk assessment consideration at each outpatient visit.
- For hospitalized patients, document risk-benefit analysis each time you make a significant clinical decision, such as on admission, when changing the level of suicide precautions, and when altering "privileges."

Courts have weighed in on other factors considered important in a mental health professional's exercise of proper judgment in diagnosis and treatment of suicidal patients. One such factor is the need to respond to new information. The court in *Kerker v. Hurwitz* (1990) permitted the plaintiff to go forward with a suit against his psychiatrist, without expert testimony, for allowing him to "remain in a hospital room with the same sprinkler pipes from which he had previously attempted to hang himself." The court's displeasure regarding the failure to move the patient after his previous suicide attempt is revealed in the judge's word choice. Similarly, a physician and hospital were liable for discharging a patient on the basis of a mental status evaluation made 41 days earlier that failed to take into account the patient's subsequent seizures and assaultive behavior (*Homere v. State of New York* 1974).

Another factor in exercising proper judgment in the treatment of suicidal patients is the need to deliver care that is appropriate in light of the seriousness of the situation, regardless of the patient's ability to pay. A provider

Risk Management Issues 161

who addresses a patient's or family's concerns about payment by offering suitable treatment alternatives may be protected from liability (see, e.g., *Paddock v. Chacko* 1988), but one who appears to base treatment decisions entirely on the level of insurance coverage without providing such alternatives will have a hard time defending his or her actions (see *Tabor v. Doctors Memorial Hospital* 1990).

Providers may support their claims that they have used proper judgment by consulting with other providers, although this is not generally required. A general practitioner who referred an adult patient to a psychiatric clinic for care he deemed beyond his expertise was not found to have an additional duty to consult with these same providers before prescribing a small dose of Thorazine (*Brandt v. Grubin* 1974). From a clinical perspective, Jobes and Berman (1993) suggest that "consultation with regard to suicidal patients is especially useful in that these patients . . . often assume demanding–dependent postures in the therapeutic relationship, thus presenting frequent and intense crises" that can cause the therapist to "lose sight of the long-term issues and treatment plan" (p. 95). To the extent that consultation allows a provider to gain a fresh perspective on a patient or even on a patient/provider relationship, it can only help in the defense of a later allegation of negligence.

Duty to Warn/Duty to Maintain Patients' Confidentiality

Tarasoff v. Regents of the University of California (1974) is among the most well known decisions articulating a specific duty for mental health professionals: the duty to warn identifiable individuals who might be harmed by a patient's actions. In many states, the duty to warn coexists with the duty to maintain a patient's confidentiality, and the potential conflict can be confusing for mental health care professionals. The California Appeals Court addressed the conflict directly in the 1978 case *Bellah v. Greenson*. Finding a psychiatrist was not negligent, even though he did not warn a patient's parents about her suicidal tendencies, the court reaffirmed the importance of maintaining confidentiality, especially in the treatment of outpatients. However, the application of these duties varies by state, and mental health care professionals should familiarize themselves with the governing statutes, regulations, and cases addressing the duty to warn and the duty to maintain confidentiality in their own states. In addition, providers can consider adopting the following risk management strategies:

- Discuss the limits of confidentiality with patients and give specific examples of instances that might warrant breach of this duty.
- If appropriate, ask patients for permission to keep their family members or significant others apprised of their progress.
- Probe for a reasonable amount of detail in determining whether a patient presents a risk of harm to others who might be identifiable.

Balancing the duty to warn against the duty to maintain confidentiality may present a provider with a dilemma—a situation in which any choice might lead to some kind of lawsuit. In these circumstances, it is fair to make a decision that reflects the position you would prefer to defend.

Duty to Supervise

The duty owed by clinical supervisors to their trainees' patients, even though they may never meet face to face (O'Keeffe and O'Keeffe 1993), is little appreciated. This duty requires them to supervise their trainees and delegate responsibility in a reasonable manner. This duty may extend to patients who are never actually seen by the supervisors. In finding attending surgeons liable for inadequately supervising a resident, a Michigan court described the duty this way:

> Even though the surgical procedure was actually performed by a resident, defendants were under a duty to see that it was performed properly. It is their skill and training as specialists which fits them for that task, and their advanced learning which enables them to judge the competency of the resident's performance. (*McCullough v. Hutzel Hospital* 1979)

The duty to supervise in a reasonable manner comprises three essential elements: 1) educating trainees in accord with national standards of practice, 2) periodically evaluating their competency in light of these standards, and 3) delegating responsibility commensurate with their competency (Butters and Strope 1996). Supervisors can assume that they will be expected to maintain their own knowledge and skills at levels that reflect evolving national standards. As psychiatric training programs shift from a psychodynamic to a psychobiological focus (Rodenhauser 1992), supervisors trained in psychosocial skills may, for example, find they need to master sufficient discipline-specific skills in somatic approaches so that they will be able to educate and evaluate trainees in a manner that appropriately protects patients.

Vaguely defined or shifting reporting relationships pervade health care training programs. Feinstein (1997) has described some of the difficulty entailed:

> A different problem in supervision is the multiple layers of faculty personnel among whom responsibility can be diffused for the process of evaluation, advancement, and, if needed, remediation of house staff. The faculty personnel can include a departmental chairman, chief of the service, chief of a firm, departmental education director, residency program director, and the ad hoc attending physician. Sometimes neither the house staff nor the faculty may know which person has the most immediate or ultimate responsibility for the evaluation decisions. (p. 1288)

Training programs for mental health care professionals are subject to the same confusion, sometimes exacerbated by cross-discipline reporting relationships. To further complicate matters, professionals in one discipline who oversee advanced-level trainees in another discipline are often unclear about both supervisory authority and responsibility. As the supervision of advanced practice nurses by psychiatrists spreads increasingly through managed systems, many of the ambiguities of this relationship are likely to draw greater clinician and administrative attention.

A task force convened by the Risk Management Foundation of the Harvard Medical Institutions to draft guidelines for prescribing psychiatrists in collaborative, consultative, or supervisory relationships with other mental health providers recommends that patients, trainees, and supervisors discuss and agree on their respective roles (Sederer et al. 1998). The following are additional risk management strategies for supervisors of mental health care trainees:

- Periodically review the scope of supervision with training program directors, addressing specifically the expectations for therapists, social workers, psychologists, advanced practice nurses, psychiatrists, or others who supervise across disciplines.
- Maintain knowledge and skills that reflect advancements in the profession.
- Regularly evaluate the knowledge and skill base of supervisees, independently assessing patients if necessary.
- Implement a system to document the evaluation of supervisees.
- Delegate responsibility commensurate with supervisees' level of skill and experience.
- Remind supervisees to call for advice or assistance in treating patients as needed and refrain from chastising those who do so.

Harm

In most medical malpractice actions, a plaintiff must demonstrate that he or she has suffered some kind of physical, quantifiable harm, beyond mere emotional upset. Once some sort of physical harm is proven, the plaintiff is allowed to seek compensation for emotional damages as well. However, plaintiffs alleging breach of the duty owed to them by their mental health providers are permitted to seek compensation for emotional harm only. To hold otherwise, of course, would contradict the fundamental premise of mental health care that is directed toward the relief of emotional suffering (see, e.g., *Horak v. Biris* 1985).

Causation, Proximate Cause, and Foreseeability

Requiring a plaintiff to demonstrate that the harm he or she suffered was a foreseeable result of the alleged negligence is intended to prevent the imposition of unreasonable liability. There are few, if any, risk management lessons to be learned from the suicide cases that turn on the issue of proximate cause, except that after a suicide has occurred it generally appears more "foreseeable" than before.

Risks Particular to Managed Care

Risk of Allowing Compensation to Determine Treatment Decisions

Both providers and patients fear that provider incentives connected to the delivery of managed health care will work too effectively, causing providers to limit or withhold care that is actually necessary (Benda and Rozovsky 1998, citing Clancy and Brody 1995). In a strictly capitated environment, providers are paid at a predetermined rate based on an estimate of the cost of caring for a given number of "covered lives." Care that costs more than this amount represents a loss to the providers, whereas care costing less results in a profit. Benda and Rozovsky (1998) describe capitation as an "induce(ment) to providers to deliver only the most appropriate services in an efficient manner" (§3.3.3C). Capitation rates, rarely generous, challenge providers to deliver care in a cost-conscious manner and to use their resources wisely, including the skills of staff, colleagues, and cotreaters. Wise utilization strategies, however, can look very much like denial of care or inappropriate reduction of services. This becomes especially true when a tragic outcome occurs. It is easy for judges and juries to be swayed by the ostensibly logical retrospective argument that just one more action or service, particularly one that was more readily provided in the past, might have prevented a bad outcome. Therefore, mental health professionals who treat suicidal patients while in an environment where cost-containment measures have been implemented should take extra care and may consider adopting some of the following risk management strategies:

- Use caution when switching from services provided by real people to those provided by automated equipment. If a change is being made from a telephone answering service to an answering machine, call the machine regularly to collect messages and ensure that it works properly. If patients' medical records are being computerized, keep hard-copy backups until the system runs without glitches.
- When duties are being reassigned from clinical to nonclinical staff, assess the risks and benefits of the changes *before and after* implementation.
- When you are supervising advanced practice nurses with prescribing privileges, ensure that you are not telling the nurses one thing (e.g., "Call me if you have any questions"), while acting in a way that undermines that instruction (e.g., ignoring pages or admonishing the supervisees for interrupting you).

The need to deal with financial issues in mental health care is not new. The pressures of capitation echo the concerns providers have felt for decades, concerns about costs exceeding expenses. A case involving the death of a mentally ill patient who leaped from a hospital window, decided in 1891, articulated the rule that hospitals and physicians are required to exercise due care to all patients, not care apportioned to the amount of money the patient agrees to pay. Paupers and millionaires are owed the same duty (*Harris v. Woman's Hospital* 1891). This principle may seem easy enough for the court to determine, but it sets a hard standard to live by when the service to society of treating the most seriously ill patients may be "rewarded" with financial loss.

As the *Harris* case illustrates, concerns about financial risk to mental health care providers preceded the advent of managed care. However, managed care has reintroduced both the concept and the reality of financial risk to providers who have been largely protected from it by third-party payers, usually insurance companies. The more recent case of *Tabor v. Doctors Memorial Hospital* (1990) highlights the decision-making process of a psychiatrist who, upon realizing that insurance might not cover the hospitalization he proposed for a suicidal patient, changed his mind and recommended instead that the patient go home to be closely watched by his parents. The patient's subsequent suicide precipitated a lawsuit in which both the psychiatrist and the physician organization that employed him were deemed negligent. It is entirely possible that the psychiatrist's initial decision to hospitalize was hastily made and deserved the reconsideration sparked by the insurance issue. However, the record did not reflect a risk-benefit analysis regarding hospitalization of the patient, and the family and hospital staff clearly associated the changed plan with the possible lack of coverage.

It is not clear how far courts will go in holding mental health care professionals responsible for rendering treatment that is unlikely to be remunerated. Providers who treat suicidal patients risk provoking claims of abandonment if they attempt to protect themselves from financial loss by terminating treatment of patients who are in crisis.

The court in *Wilson v. Blue Cross of Southern California* (1990) indicated that some of the burden of responsibility carried by mental health professionals who treat suicidal patients may be shared by insurers whose utilization review staff approve or deny coverage for patients. In *Wilson* a depressed patient was hospitalized for drug dependency and anorexia. His treating physician recommended 3–4 weeks of inpatient care, but the Blue Cross utilization reviewers authorized only a 10-day stay. Discharged after 10 days, the patient committed suicide, and the court permitted the patient's estate to sue the insurance company under a theory of joint and several liability. The matter was settled after that decision and before trial on the merits of the case.

Although managed care organizations could be held liable following the *Wilson* reasoning, this possibility has not blossomed in the climate of ERISA preemptions granted to managed care organizations. ERISA, the Employee Retirement Income Security Act of 1974, is a federal statute intended to protect employees' retirement funds from being chipped away by endless lawsuits. The statue has been extended to include employee benefit funds, such as health care benefit funds, protecting managed care organizations from liability for decisions made "in the context of making a determination about the availability of benefits under the plan" (*Corcoran v. United HealthCare* 1992). Although ERISA preemption is facing vigorous challenges, it currently continues to shield managed care organizations from liability in many cases, therefore making individual providers more likely defendants in neg-

Risk Management Issues

ligence actions. Essentially, providers may represent a patient's sole possible source of compensation.

Capitation and the threat of not receiving payment for services rendered represent one type of financial incentive, but there are others that mental health care providers must also identify and address. *Withholds* are such an additional concern; although in reality they represent a percentage of payments owed to providers that is held back by the payor and reearned by the provider for meeting predetermined goals, they can look suspiciously like bonuses awarded to groups of providers who have complied with an insuror's incentives. Although such incentives may incorporate patient satisfaction data and quality measurements such as hospital readmittance rates, they are generally profit-driven goals.

Clinicians working in managed systems should acquaint themselves fully with the existence of such carrot-and-stick incentives and apply risk management strategies to provider/managed care contract negotiations in one or more of the following ways:

- Read all managed care contracts carefully. If you lack the required time or expertise, delegate this task to a knowledgeable, responsible associate or lawyer.
- Do not enter into unrealistic capitated agreements. Thoroughly assess and document the costs of treatment in the system. Bargaining downward from an artificially low number can promote financial disaster.
- Look for incentives that reward patient satisfaction and delivery of quality care, not just increased profits. In the treatment of suicidal patients, for example, participate in developing outcome measures that appropriately define quality care.
- Look for incentives that spread financial risk among a moderately sized group of providers and patients. The group should be large enough so that the financial risk of treating a small number of high-cost, suicidal patients will not unduly influence individual treatment decisions, but small enough for providers to maintain accountability for reaching both quality and cost-containment goals.
- Ascertain that the managed care organizations you contract with support disclosure of general financial incentives to patients.
- If care you recommend for a patient is denied by the managed care organization or declined by the patient for financial reasons, take action commensurate with the level of risk involved to the patient or others. Patients you deem at high risk may need to be hospitalized while you continue negotiations.

- Follow the proper appeals process. Ask to have the case reviewed by a specialist in your field, and be clear about the specific facts that have informed your treatment recommendation. Your rationale, not your conclusion, will help you make a persuasive argument. When possible, distinguish this case from apparently similar but less serious cases and compare it with cases with adverse outcomes. The Wickline case (Wickline v. State 1986), in which a provider was found liable for failing to appeal a decision to limit care, provides a warning to clinicians who might too readily accept denial of a patient's requested benefits.
- Consider and discuss alternative treatment options with the patient (or the patient's family, as appropriate). If you undertake a different course of action than originally planned, document the risk-benefit analysis that led to this decision.
- When appropriate, offer to refer the patient to sources of free care or reduced-fee care, and facilitate transfer of information to the new provider, as appropriate, if the patient chooses this option.
- Consider buying insurance for catastrophic financial losses—often called stop-loss insurance—so that a bad year will not drive you out of business.
- Find out whether the terms of your managed care contracts are negotiable. If so, assign negotiations to a knowledgeable, responsible person who has read the contracts thoroughly.
- Consider preparing information to be distributed to patients that suggests possible actions they can take if coverage is denied. Suggestions may be as simple as the following:

  > Carefully review all documents, brochures, letters, and fliers from your managed care company. These should explain your medical and mental health benefits. If you receive your health benefits through your job, ask your employer for help in understanding any information that is not clear. Someone in Human Resources should be able to explain your health care benefits to you and help you contact your insurance company if there is a misunderstanding. When there is a disagreement regarding services that are covered, send a letter to your insurance company or managed care organization explaining what you want and why you think they should pay for it. Keep a copy for yourself.

- Beware of contractual termination clauses. As initially conceptualized, these served to allow either the provider or the managed care organization to terminate its agreement for any reason, or no reason at all, with relatively short notice, usually 90 days. As health care delivery systems have responded to public pressure to measure, report, and compare outcomes, the providers have grown to fear termination of contracts on the basis of being labeled an "outlier" who incurs excessive costs within a managed care organization. A factor that raises the stakes is the provider's awareness that seldom is only one contract at stake, since most managed care organizations require providers to reveal terminations from other contracts, which might initiate termination of other managed care contracts.

- Request contracts that are renewed annually, otherwise terminable only for cause.
- Support the creation of independent managed care appeal boards empowered to resolve patient coverage issues in a timely manner.
- Promote the adoption of practice guidelines promulgated by respected groups of health care professionals, such as national medical associations, to ensure that overall quality of care continues to improve.
- Support legislative action that limits managed care organizations' ability to terminate providers for reasons that contravene public policy.
- Consider joining a professional guild or union to promote the values that you believe define your profession (Roemer 1998).

Informed Consent in the Managed Care Environment

The principles of informed consent apply equally whether treatment occurs in fee-for-service or managed care environments. Although some managed care organizations denied any intention of curbing providers' ability to engage patients in meaningful consent discussions, they also included clauses in their provider contracts prohibiting discussion of matters that might promote dissatisfaction among patients. Such prohibitions, dubbed by the popular media "gag clauses," were subsequently brought to public awareness and ultimately removed or invalidated by state laws. Providers are, therefore, presumed to be free to discuss any and all treatment options with patients, even treatments not covered by their health plans. Mental health care providers should be aware, however, that both a healthy degree of paternalism and the natural desire not to attract attention to one's practice may curb a provider's willingness to engage patients in discussions of treatment options not covered by their insurers. The strategies for dealing with informed consent issues that involve suicidal patients treated in a managed care environment are the same as those appropriate to the fee-for-service environment:

- Discuss the risks and benefits of treatment options.
- Address specific risks that might be of particular concern to the patient,

such as side effects of medication that have proved intolerable to the patient in the past.
- Come to an agreement with the patient (or the person qualified to make health care decisions on the patient's behalf) regarding a treatment plan.
- Remember that patients who are not otherwise deemed incompetent are free to change their minds and refuse treatment at any time. A patient's choice of an unpleasant or unwise course of action is not, in itself, evidence of incompetence to make treatment decisions.
- Pursue guardianship for chronically or acutely suicidal patients who are incompetent to make informed health care decisions.

Conclusion

As noted initially, clinicians cannot treat suicidal patients without exposing themselves to risk. Managed care introduces potential aids to treatment along with other factors that increase clinicians' exposure to liability. A managed system that emphasizes teamwork and coordinated care may conceivably provide superior care, and clinicians who are aware of the elements of risk associated with treatment will be more likely to address the needs of their suicidal patients while avoiding excessive exposure to liability.

References

Abille v United States, 482 F Supp 703 (ND Cal 1980)

Annotation, Liability of Doctor, Psychiatrist, or Psychologist for Failure to Take Steps to Prevent Patient's Suicide, 17 ALR4th 1128 (1998)

Annotation, Malpractice Liability With Respect to Diagnosis and Treatment of Mental Disease, 99 ALR 2d 599 (1997)

Bell v New York City Health & Hospitals Corp., 90 AD2d 270 (1982)

Bellah v Greenson, 81 Cal App 3d 614 (1978)

Benda C, Rozovsky F: Liability and Risk Management in Managed Care. Gaithersburg, MD, Aspen, 1998

Brandt v Grubin, 329 A2d 82 (NJ Super 1974)

Brandvain v Ridgeview Institute, Inc., 372 SE2d 265 (Ga Ct App 1988), aff'd 382 SE2d 596 (Ga 1989)

Brennan T, Leape LL, Laird NM, et al: Incidence of adverse events and negligence in hospitalized patients: results of the Harvard Medical Practice Study I. N Engl J Med 324:370–376, 1991

Brytan H, Davis O: Managing behavioral health risks: claims analysis and risk management considerations. Vantage Point 2(2):2–5, 1997 [CNA HealthPro Publications]

Butters J, Strope J: Legal standards of conduct for students and residents: implications for health professions educators. Acad Med 71:583–590, 1996

Central Anesthesia Associates, P.C. v Worthy, 333 SE2d 829 (Ga 1985)

Clancy C, Brody H: Managed care: Jekyll or Hyde? (comment; editorial) JAMA 273:338–339, 1995

Cohen v State of NewYork, 51 AD2d 494 (1976)

Corcoran v United HealthCare, 965 F2d 1321 (5th Cir), cert denied, 16 EBC 1432 (1992)

Employee Retirement Income Security Act of 1974, Pub L No 93-406, 88 Stat 829, codified as amended at 29 USC 1001 et seq (1994)

Farwell v Un, 902 F2d 282 (4th Cir 1990)

Feinstein A: System, supervision, standards, and the 'epidemic' of negligent medical errors (commentary). Arch Intern Med 157:1285–1289, 1997

Gregory v Robinson, 338 SW2d 88 (Mo 1960)

Gutheil T: The wellsprings of litigation, in The Mental Health Practitioner and the Law. Edited by Lifson L, Simon R. Cambridge, MA, Harvard University Press, 1998, pp 250–261

Harris v Woman's Hospital, 14 NYS 881 (1891)

Helling v Carey, 519 P2d 981 (Wash 1974)

Helms L, Helms C: Forty years of litigation involving residents and their training, II: Malpractice issues. Acad Med 66:718–725, 1991

Homere v State of New York, 361 NYS2d 820 (1974)

Horak v Biris, 474 NE2d 13 (Ill App 1985)

Huntley v State, 464 NE2d 467 (NY 1984)

Jobes D, Berman A: Suicide and malpractice liability: assessing and revising policies, procedures, and practice in outpatient settings. Professional Psychology: Research and Practice 24:91–99, 1993

Kerker v Hurwitz, 163 AD2d 859 (1990)

Liability for Patient Suicide. Arlington, VA, Psychiatrists' Purchasing Group, 1994

McCullough v Hutzel Hospital, 276 NW2d 569 (Mich Ct App 1979)

O'Keeffe R, O'Keeffe C: Becoming brother's keeper: legal responsibilities of those supervising care by residents. N C Med J 54:166–168, 1993

Packman WL, Harris EA: Legal issues and risk management in suicidal patients, in Risk Management With Suicidal Patients. Edited by Bongar B, Berman AL, Maris RW. New York, Guilford, 1998, pp 150–186

Paddock v Chacko, 552 So2d 410 (Fla Dist Ct App 1988), review denied, 553 So2d 168 (Fla 1989)

ProMutual Group Risk Management Overview 1987–1996. Psychiatry: A Risk Management Analysis. Boston, MA, ProMutual Group, 1997

Rodenhauser P: Psychiatry residency programs: trends in psychotherapy supervision. Am J Psychother 46:240–249, 1992

Roemer J: Fighting back: how labor unions are helping physicians regain some of their lost power. Hippocrates, April 1998, pp 50–59

Sederer L, Ellison J, Keyes C: Guidelines for prescribing psychiatrists in consultative, collaborative, and supervisory relationships. Psychiatr Serv 49:1197–1202, 1998

Sheeley v Memorial Hospital, 710 A2d 161 (RI 1998)

Simon R: Clinical Psychiatry and the Law, 2nd Edition. Washington, DC, American Psychiatric Press, 1992

Tabor v Doctors Memorial Hospital, 563 So2d 233 (La 1990)

Tarasoff v Regents of the University of California, 551 P2d 334 (1974)

Timmins v State, 296 NYS2d 429 (1968)

Wickline v State, 192 Cal App 3d 1630 (1986)

Wilkinson A: Psychiatric malpractice, in Medical Malpractice, Vol 2. Edited by Louisell D, Williams H. San Francisco, CA, Matthew Bender, 1998, pp 17A-1–17A-211

Wilson v Blue Cross of Southern California, 222 Cal App 3d 660 (1990)

Zaremski M, Goldstein L: Medical and Hospital Negligence, Vols 1–4. Deerfield, IL, Callaghan & Company, 1988–1990 [updated with pocket parts through 1990]

CHAPTER 9

In the Aftermath of Suicide: Needs and Interventions

Steve Stelovich, M.D.

Completed suicide is all too grim a reality in society and in health care, yet suggestions for addressing the problems that emerge subsequent to a suicide are few and far between. Of 1,500 recent articles on suicide, I found only a handful of titles that address both postsuicide sequelae and recommendations for handling them. Even fewer offer a structured or comprehensive approach to dealing with postsuicide issues (Bartles 1987; Bengesser 1988; Chance 1988; Cooper 1995; Cotton et al. 1983; Dunne-Maxim et al. 1992; Hodgkinson 1987; Kaye and Soreff 1991; Litman 1965; Neill et al. 1974; Stelovich 1997).

The enormous literature devoted to suicide focuses almost exclusively on epidemiology, etiology, and prevention. Because suicide marks the end of a health care provider's relationship with a patient, it is understandable that our clinical literature focuses more readily on the issues relevant to the living patient. Anyone who has had to deal with the aftermath of suicide, however, recognizes the complexity and seriousness of the needs of those who survive. This chapter attempts to fill a void in the literature on suicide by providing a framework for identifying and responding to the needs that emerge in the wake of a suicide.

Over the past 25 years, I have participated in or conducted more than 100 suicide reviews. In doing so, I have interviewed the clinicians who were providing treatment, the bereaved family members and friends, and the other patients who were touched by the deaths that occurred in institutional settings. In addition, I have coordinated or participated in institutional or administrative responses to patient deaths. Over time, I have recognized a common set of problems that emerge among each of these affected groups. The paradigm I developed for identifying and managing these problems has proven useful in a variety of ways and in many different settings. It has served to provide a structure for understanding the different ways in which a person's suicide casts its shadow over the lives of others. It has also provided a template for planning responses at all levels, from individual to institutional and societal. Perhaps most importantly, I have used it to predict potential problems among the survivors of a suicide, allowing early intervention and preventive action. In this chapter, I explain this paradigm and illustrate it with an example that draws on details of several actual cases, disguised sufficiently to ensure anonymity.

A Model for the Management of a Completed Suicide: Four Groups and Four Tasks

In the aftermath of suicide, who is affected and in what ways? What tasks must be undertaken to deal with their immediate and longer-term needs? These are the key questions that must be answered if one is to manage the problems that most commonly emerge when a person takes his or her own life. Surprisingly, the answers to these questions are quite straightforward.

Four groups of people within the patient's universe are most significantly affected by suicide: clinicians and other professionals directly responsible for the deceased person's care; bereaved family and close friends; patients and other individuals who were part of the deceased's treatment cohort; and the medical, civil, or institutional authorities who were indirectly but meaningfully responsible for the deceased person's well-being.

For every death through suicide, at least several family members' or friends' lives are affected. Given the greater prevalence of suicide among individuals with a positive family history for suicide, some surviving family members will ultimately experience multiple traumatic losses. Help for family and friends may be available from their religious organizations, if they are affiliated with one, or from secular organizations such as the American Foundation for Suicide Prevention, which runs groups for those bereaved by suicide. For a variety of reasons, the family and friends of a person who commits suicide may also seek contact with the deceased's treatment system. Such contact arises, for example, when those closest to the person who committed suicide seek to understand more fully why the suicide occurred. At other times, family members seek former treaters angrily in an effort to determine and assign blame for a devastating loss. The death of a loved one, for others, may become an opportunity for life review and a decision to seek treatment.

Suicide touches the majority of mental health clinicians in one way or another. Twenty percent of psychologists and 50% of psychiatrists can expect to lose a patient to suicide. One-sixth of individuals who complete suicide are, at the time of their death, engaged in a psychotherapy. Primary care clinicians, too, experience the loss of patients through suicide. Many of the patients who complete suicide saw a physician (who was often a primary care physician) within the preceding weeks (Fawcett et al. 1993; Roy 1982). Medical school and residency training offer little or no preparation for dealing with the sequelae of suicide. Clinicians who have experienced the suicide of a patient, however, are often deeply affected. After losing a patient in this way, a clinician may subsequently avoid treating suicidal patients, may even choose to change professions, or may approach the care of future suicidal patients with anxiety that interferes with clinical judgment.

Patients sharing treatment resources constitute a potentially neglected group of those affected by a suicide. When a member of a psychotherapy group completes a suicide, for example, the other members are forced to confront painful issues. They will wonder whether they played any role in the death or could have played a role in rescue. They may question the efficacy of a treatment that has failed to prevent a death, or they may renew their determination to participate in treatment in the hope of avoiding a similar outcome. Even beyond the other members of a defined psychotherapy group, word of a suicide may spread to others in a vaguely defined community of patients. Individuals who were hospitalized at the same time may have stayed informally in touch, telephoning each other in times of crisis or engaging in various types of friendships. Persons in such informally associated connections may share the loss even though they no longer are connected with the formerly shared treatment resources. When the connection with treatment is not current, supports for healthy coping may be limited, heightening the risks of imitative suicide or other types of acting-out behavior.

Members of a further group constitute an additional, often unrecognized, faction of those affected by a suicide. The medical, institutional, or civil authorities indirectly but meaningfully responsible for a patient's care and safety can find themselves in the very midst of the difficulties stirred up by a patient's death. Unlike the inpatient attending psychiatrist or case manager or the outpatient psychotherapist who has directly cared for a patient, these authorities may be swept up into the complications of a suicide without having ever met or personally provided care to the deceased patient. In the hospital setting, the chief of a psychiatry department and the administrator of the hospital occupy roles vulnerable to such involvements. Though perhaps removed from the direct care of the deceased, they are frequently named in malpractice claims that arise following suicides attributed to negligent treatment. At even further remove, though involved from time to time, are such groups as the boards of registration for the professionals involved, professional societies, or the police. In defining the members of this group, it is sufficient to ask, "Who is indirectly but so *closely* enough involved in the death at hand that one might reasonably expect him or her to be affected in some way?"

From the perspective of the clinical setting, then, we can conveniently refer to the four major groups of people affected by a suicide as family, clinicians, other patients, and administrators. For the sake of simplicity, these terms will be employed through the rest of the chapter. The use of these terms, however, should not be taken to imply rigid or precise definitions of the groups' boundaries. The boundaries, in reality, may be difficult to determine. Membership in one of the four groups, moreover, does not eliminate the possibility of membership in one of the other groups as well.

Among the tasks that confront members of these four groups affected by suicide, four basic processes have crucial roles. I refer to them as anticipating, announcing, assisting, and assessing. The permutations determined by a matrix of the four groups and four processes is demonstrated in Figure 9–1. In such a grid, each box represents the single task being undertaken by one of the involved groups (examples of such tasks are shown in the figure). The complete display, all 16 boxes, can be understood as the full complement of activities that must be successfully addressed for there to be a satisfactory outcome. This matrix organizes the tasks that follow a suicide without, however, prescribing specific interventions. Each component cell in the matrix requires that the clinician evaluate, diagnose (in the original sense of developing a thorough understanding of), and formulate appropriate interventions. I will illustrate the components of this matrix, which constitutes a paradigm for the successful management of many of the needs that emerge following a completed suicide. After I define each process, I will illustrate it with reference to the following composite case vignette.[1]

---

[1] The author wishes to thank this book's editor, Dr. Ellison, for his assistance in developing this illustrative vignette.

	Anticipating	Announcing	Assisting	Assessing
Family	A physician openly discusses the likelihood of death in the context of current treatment.	A mental health provider gives information regarding the death to family members as soon as possible.	A family member who becomes depressed after a suicide is provided treatment.	A family is met with 1 year after the death of a member to "set things to rest."
Clinicians	Contingencies for handling the death of specific patients are made.	Clinicians on an inpatient unit meet to hear and share information regarding a patient's death.	A clinician who begins to doubt his own ability to provide good care is counseled by a peer.	A suicide is formally reviewed and ward policies are changed in view of the findings.
Patients	Suicide precautions for specific patients are reviewed with others.	Facts regarding the death of a patient are shared in a unit meeting of patients.	A patient who evidences a psychotic belief that he caused the death is treated.	A patient reviews current policies on readmission to a unit where a suicide previously occurred.
Administration	Serious suicide risk is conveyed to the medical director or a unit.	Facts about a suicide are quickly conveyed to a hospital medical director and administrator.	A hospital administrator is assisted in preparing a statement to the press regarding the suicide of a patient in the facility.	A health providing organization regularly reviews the results of clinical suicide reviews to determine whether policies or facilities should be reconfigured.

FIGURE 9–1. Management matrix and intervention examples.

Case Example

Julie, a 24-year-old woman diagnosed with schizoaffective disorder, lived independently in an apartment and worked several hours each weekday at the Salvation Army thrift shop. Julie received medications from a psychiatrist (Dr. P.) and attended biweekly supportive psychotherapy sessions with a social worker (Ms. T.). In the past, Julie had responded to painful disappointments with suicidal ideation. On one occasion, she had even taken a small overdose, enough medication to make her sleepy and nauseated, before she decided to call her psychotherapist, who sent an ambulance to Julie's apartment so that she could be assessed in the emergency room.

Anticipating

Anticipating, the first of the tasks that help us cope with the aftermath of a suicide, is the only one that begins to occur even prior to the patient's death. Anticipation is the "giving of advance thought, discussion, or treatment" (*Webster's Seventh New Collegiate Dictionary* 1963, p. 38). Anticipation is the process that will later be invoked when family, clinicians, patients, and authorities all ask, "What could have been done differently?" Many patients who ultimately die through suicide will have previously revealed suicidal ideation, discussed their plans, or even threatened their care providers and/or significant others with this possibility. A clinician who recognizes a patient's potential for self-destruction could respond in any number of ways, including serially assessing and documenting the patient's degree of suicidality, formulation of a "no suicide contract" (see Chapters 1 and 8, this volume, for discussion of the pitfalls of this strategy), intensifying treatment by increasing the frequency of individual or group treatment sessions by adding telephone check-ins, or admitting the patient to a more protective treatment setting such as a partial hospital program, acute residential treatment facility, or full hospitalization.

In the aftermath of a suicide, this anticipatory component of treatment takes on a central importance. Though the patient's life has ended, the clinician will be able to minimize the experience of guilt and remorse by knowing that adequate and appropriate treatment planning had taken place. Family members and friends who recognized that suicide was a possibility will be able to grieve their loss more effectively. Other patients who already understood how close their cohort was to suicide may be able to face the death with sadness rather than with a sense of outrage and shock that could undermine their faith in treatment. Authorities who have remained alert in a more general sense to the possibility of a suicide will have designed their treatment facilities to promote safety and maximize the likelihood of suicide prevention.

Case Example *(continued)*

When Julie learned that her mother had been diagnosed with a potentially fatal breast cancer, she experienced shock and outrage that soon gave way to despair. Julie told her psychotherapist that she would be unable to bear her mother's suffering and unwilling to bear her mother's loss. Rather than experience these, she would kill herself. She knew which over-the-counter medication to take in order to produce a fatal overdose and had obtained a large bottle as her "insurance policy."

Ms. T. responded to Julie's revelations in a variety of ways, anticipating the possibility of suicide and revising her treatment approach accordingly. At each session, she carefully assessed Julie's acute suicide risk, taking note of any changes in Julie's reports of her mother's illness and inquiring empathically but directly about suicidal thoughts or behaviors. Because Julie was having difficulty coping with her new role as an occasional caregiver, Ms. T. encouraged her to become involved in a local peer support group that helped individuals adjust to the stresses of caring for a seriously ill parent. Emergency telephone support lines and other avenues for immediate help were discussed, and Ms. T. let Julie know how to reach her for check-in discussions between their scheduled sessions. Ms. T. also prepared a written agreement or "promise" listing the ways that Julie would go about obtaining help in the event that her suicidal urges became severe [see Chapter 1, this volume, for discussion of risks of sole reliance on contracts]. Psychotherapist and patient signed this agreement, each kept a copy, and they reviewed it together periodically. Finally, Ms. T. included Dr. P. in the discussions about suicide so that he could also address these concerns with Julie and consider whether a change in the pharmacotherapy treatment plan was indicated.

As her mother's cancer and the debilitating therapeutic process progressed over a period of months, Julie continued to experience suicidal thoughts and urges that were effectively dealt with by the agreement and treatment plan, reinforced by intermittent brief overnight stays in an "observation bed." A few family meetings were incorporated into Julie's treatment, and the possibility of Julie's suicide was discussed openly. In the weeks following Julie's mother's death, all aspects of treatment were intensified, but Julie's grief was inconsolable. She was admitted to an inpatient unit and placed on 15-minute checks as an antisuicide precaution. When Julie hung herself in her hospital room, between checks, her care providers were devastated but not entirely taken off guard. They had been fully aware of the mounting suicide risk and had responded in the ways that usually prevent such a sad outcome. Though unable to prevent Julie's suicide, they had anticipated it and responded in a variety of appropriate ways.

Julie's family, too, were grief-stricken but not completely surprised. At the family meetings, Ms. T. had made certain that they understood the degree of risk associated with Julie's illness, the stress she was experiencing related to mother's cancer, and her intermittently severe urges to end her own life. The surviving family members, father and two brothers, were grateful to have been able to anticipate Julie's feelings and risk in a way that allowed them partially to prepare themselves for the subsequent events.

When Julie's support group learned of her death, the shock was mitigated by their earlier awareness that Julie's ability to deal with her mother's disease and death was complicated by her own mental illness. Julie had spoken, in the group, of her urges toward suicide. The group's leader, in fact, had on several occasions called Ms. T. to let her know how concerned the group members were about Julie's safety. Though each group member was engaged in coping with the other painful situations that had brought them there, the group was able to discuss and process Julie's suicide.

The hospital ward where Julie had hung herself was a new facility, carefully designed to minimize the risk of self-destruction. Safety concerns had mandated the adoption of many features designed for patient safety, but the possibility that Julie would hang herself with a looped up sheet attached to the ceiling light fixture had not been anticipated. The ingenuity of this method and the carefulness of Julie's timing came as a surprise to the unit director and to the hospital administration.

Announcing

The next task, in the aftermath of suicide, is what I refer to as *announcing*. To announce means "to make known publicly" (*Webster's Seventh New Collegiate Dictionary* 1963, p. 36). Family, clinicians, patients, and authorities all need to know "what really happened" as they cope with a suicide. The very way in which information is acknowledged and disseminated can have a decided impact on the consequences of this news. Was the death openly acknowledged and discussed? Was it learned about via the public media, and if so, were sufficient accurate and appropriate details shared? Or, was the matter shrouded in cloak of mystery and referred to by innuendo? The role of the health care provider in announcing or providing information can be crucial in how this information is received, understood, and acted on. Clinicians need to know the most comprehensive version of the suicide, including technical and specific detail of the events, that will allow them to provide appropriate information to others in the chain of communication. Family members often have many questions about the reasons for the suicide, painfulness of the death, or the existence of any final communication. They are prone to think of new questions as days go by, so they should be encouraged to bring up concerns that emerge following an initial discussion. Other patients may focus on the danger signs that they observed but pushed out of their awareness or the now regrettable promise to share a secret that, if divulged, might have prevented a death. Authorities must in addition attend to information that will aid in risk management, such as errors in the treatment protocol or documentation of treatment. In this way, they can increase the protection of other patients and prepare to respond to any claims of negligence.

Case Example *(continued)*

When Julie's hanging was discovered by the nurse performing checks, she was immediately cut down from her makeshift noose and resuscitation was attempted but was not successful. The unit director was notified, and she telephoned Ms. T. and Dr. P. to discuss the details of Julie's death. These outpatient clinicians were later grateful to have received complete and timely notification of Julie's suicide, which allowed them to begin assimilating and adjusting to this unfortunate outcome.

In discussion with the unit director, Ms. T. volunteered to notify Julie's surviving family members and support group of her death, given her ongoing relationship with them. She notified Julie's father and brother immediately by telephone and scheduled a family meeting for discussion early the next day. At that meeting, she expressed her condolences and discussed the details of Julie's death. Ms. T. was less detailed in her call to the support group's leader but announced Julie's death and discussed treatment resources that would be available for any group members who experienced a need to process Julie's death in a setting even more supportive than that provided by the group. The group leader, in turn, brought the news to the other group members, paving the way for discussion. The unit director took responsibility for notifying the hospital's risk management director, administrator, and medical director. These hospital personnel were thereby prepared to receive and respond to subsequent questions from the medical examiner's office. In this way, all the involved groups of individuals became aware of the suicide and obtained information that was accurate, timely, and sufficiently detailed. In all these communications, an attempt was made to respect the family's privacy by limiting communication to only the information that was necessary.

Assisting

I use the term *assisting* to refer to the giving of support and aid (*Webster's Seventh Collegiate Dictionary* 1963, p. 52) that helps family, clinicians, patients, and authorities cope with the immediate crises that occur in the wake of a suicide. Once the involved clinicians have been notified of a suicide, they need to notify appropriate other parties very promptly. Their own needs, however, should not be neglected. The involved clinicians should be offered an opportunity to debrief and address the feelings that inevitably accompany the death of a patient. Sadness over the loss of a human life; guilt over any perceived shortcomings in the treatment; and anger at being exposed to professional scrutiny, criticism, and liability will weave through the clinician's thoughts. The availability of an empathic colleague, an experienced administrator, a close friend or partner, or a psychotherapist may facilitate the clinician's adjustment to the suicide. A "suicide review" or "psychological autopsy" often provides support as well. Some clinicians, unfortunately, have no opportunity to discuss their reactions to this type of event, and they may subsequently avoid suicidal patients or treat them with excessive caution or control.

Family members' needs are often the most excrutiating and acute. Even the acceptance of the suicide may present a painful challenge. Sometimes it is even difficult for family members to believe that their relative's death was self-inflicted rather than accidental or homicidal. Once the death has been accepted and the nature of the death is understood, a storm of feelings will affect the family. Grief, surprise, rage, loneliness, and a wish to assign blame are all likely to appear in the course of coping with a suicide. Clinicians or others who aid the surviving family members of a suicide may help them by letting them tell their story, reminiscing about the deceased, empathizing with their emotional reactions, helping them deal with the concrete aspects of funeral planning, and pointing them toward useful resources such as the many sincere and helpful books on survivors (Bolton 1983; Fine 1997; Hewett 1980).

Other patients emerge with a variety of needs in the wake of a cohort's suicide. One might experience a powerful reduction in her own suicidal urges, recognizing how real the loss will be and how devastating the consequences. Another, by contrast, may become even more self-destructive, deriving instruction on "how to succeed" from the event.

Commonly, a fellow patient will claim, "You may not think that I'm responsible, but I'm sure I could have prevented it if I'd only talked with him." On occasion, another patient will reveal that he had been scheduled to call or meet with the deceased at the time when the suicide occurred. Other patients may experience obsessive or delusional feelings of responsibility, such as a fear that an "evil thought" about the patient led to the suicide.

Authorities' needs for assistance are varied. For the administrator of a public hospital vying for funding, a suicide could be construed as "proof positive" that services in the hospital are poor and that funding should be discontinued or moved elsewhere. In slightly varied circumstances, the same suicide might be used by the hospital to support requests for increased funding aimed at improving the quality of service. The medical director of a unit on which several suicides have occurred could be confronted with reviews or investigations of circumstances on the part of contracting agencies. The specifics differ in each instance. Administrators, however, will be generally called on to certify that they have exercised appropriate oversight in the spe-

In the Aftermath of Suicide

cific case and that they can guarantee the safety of other individuals for whom they are responsible. The care must be reviewed, the patient's behavior must be understood, and the completeness of documentation must be ascertained. Assistance in this process can have significant impact on systems of service delivery.

Case Example *(continued)*

When Ms. T. spoke with Julie's father and brother, she noted quickly that both were overwhelmed with what had become a double loss. Father appeared numbed with grief, though superficially he continued to cope effectively with the demands of his role. His questions were largely of a procedural nature as he sought to manage Julie's cremation and estate. He willingly accepted the name of a local organization that ran "survivor groups" for the bereaved. Julie's brother, on the other hand, appeared to be quite severely depressed. Though he expressed grateful recognition of the ways in which the hospital had tried to help Julie, he was clearly on the verge of decompensating. Ms. T. arranged for him to attend a partial hospital day program, where he received counseling and was started on an antidepressant in a safe, protective environment.

Ms. T.'s discussion with the leader of Julie's group helped the leader understand that Julie's suicide had nothing to do with either the group or any behavior of the group's members. This made it more possible to allay the group members' guilty feelings and speculations and help them engage with one another in confronting their new and unwelcome loss. The group leader brought several books about suicide and survivors to the group so that members could receive additional support through reading of others' experiences in this realm.

The unit director and hospital administrator were initially mortified by the news that a suicide had occurred despite a secure treatment setting, a well-constructed treatment plan, and an ostensibly safe environment. Their faith in the safety and security of their treatment facility had been shaken. Discussions with the hospital risk management division, however, served to remind them that careful consideration had been given to safety issues in the construction of the unit. Expert consultation had been sought and the unit had been planned by taking into account the very highest of community standards. They were reminded that no place can be rendered entirely safe. These conversations helped reduce anxiety on the part of the hospital administrator and unit director. They freed up energy to focus on the tasks at hand. In addition, a tone of continuous quality improvement was set, aiding in the later assessment phase of work that looked to the future.

Finally, Julie's inpatient clinicians and her outpatient psychotherapist and pharmacotherapist were able to address their own reactions to the death once others were sufficiently attended to. Ms. T. had lost another patient through suicide, had admitted Julie for protection, and had to confront considerable anger at the hospital for allowing Julie to be unobserved even for 15 minutes at a time, which the inpatient staff had considered an acceptable level of risk. Dr. P. had to cope with a sense of failure and powerlessness that was very distressing as he recognized how unable he had been to prevent Julie's death.

Assessing

The concluding process in coping with suicide's aftermath is what I call *assessing,* a term that denotes an assignment of importance to the event (*Webster's Seventh Collegiate Dictionary* 1963, p. 53). Generally, and often at a much later time, the suicide is assessed and reviewed in a more analytic fashion. Such review often leads to a change in perception of the death and a fresh view of the larger "social" or "philosophical" implications. The question becomes less and less Who was responsible for this miscarriage of treatment? and more What has this death taught us about our lives?

Clinicians who successfully assess the meaning of a suicide are better able to continue treating other suicidal patients with less need for denial or overconcern. Family members may find themselves growing closer as they agree to put the deceased to rest and "go on living" rather than continuing to review and mourn the death. Other patients may in time reestablish hopefulness about their own treatments. They, too, must let their loss move from a central focus as they resume work on the problems that brought them into treatment. Authorities can use the opportunity of assessing to reflect on the meaning of a suicide and review the policies and procedures that govern treatment in their organizations. In this way, the care of future suicidal patients can be improved.

Case Example *(continued)*

Julie's psychiatrist, Dr. P., took her death very hard. Feeling a lack of anyone with whom to discuss his reactions, he instead avoided coping and found himself moving over time further away from direct patient care as he accepted increasing administrative challenges. In subsequent years, he reported, "I had no one who could help me through it, and I'd never had a suicide before. There just wasn't a way to talk about such things, and they sure tear you apart. In retrospect, I'm not sure that I would have divorced myself so radically from direct care if I could have found a way to get myself some support." Ms. T., on the other hand, had sought both the support of friends and colleagues and a brief course of psychotherapy to address the tumultuous feelings that followed her patient's suicide. In subsequent years, she found that other clinicians valued her advice on the management of patients at high risk, and she authored several papers on this topic.

Julie's family eventually felt grateful to the treatment team for the help that they had received. Julie's brother, encouraged into treatment at a relatively early stage in his depression, was able to recover fully.

The patients who had known Julie in their support group would have preferred, on the whole, not to have been forced to experience the loss of a group member by suicide. One comember, nonetheless, came to see Julie's death as a meaningful experience, one that helped her reassess her own life goals and path with helpful consequences.

The authorities at Julie's hospital assessed her death carefully and came to revise several policies in their treatment of suicidal patients. One important change was the adoption of a policy that discouraged reliance on 15-minute checks in favor of "constant observation" when suicide risk was believed to be high and patients met the criteria developed for such observation. The light fixtures were reviewed by an architectural consultant and replaced by breakaway fixtures that would not support a person's weight, should future attempts be made to use them for self-destructive behavior.

In the context of clinical management, then, the tasks that follow a suicide may be summarized as anticipating, announcing, assisting, and assessing. Anticipation in this context refers to the giving of advance thought or treatment. Announcing refers to the dissemination of information, as it becomes available, to those with appropriate need to know and permission to receive the information. Assisting is the process of lending support or assistance that may be clinical or administrative. Assessing refers to the assignment of importance and/or significance, often associated with a change in view of the suicide's meaning and a subsequent revision of treatment procedures.

In developing the above paradigm over the past 25 years, it has been my experience that interventions that might be expected to serve in all cases are difficult, if not impossible, to specify. At the same time, it has also been my experience that reasonable and helpful recommendations can almost always be made if time is spent evaluating the status of the individuals and activities contributing to the component cells of the matrix. Unanticipated clinical or emotional disturbances may be averted, and unpleasant medical-legal sequelae may be avoided.

Conclusion

A paradigm for the successful management of completed suicide requires that the clinician involved assess, understand, and develop an intervention strategy in each of 16 separate arenas (see Figure 9–1). These, in turn, are defined by a matrix of tasks (anticipating, announcing, assisting, and assessing) that need to be completed among four distinct groups (family, clinicians, patients, and administration).

Though the paradigm for handling completed suicides was developed and has been applied in clinical psychiatric settings, it would appear to lend itself to other situations in which suicide occurs, such as general medical settings, work settings, and jails and prisons. In each instance the definition of group membership must be modified, but the tasks remain unchanged. For example, in a prison setting, "clinicians," as those directly responsible for the individual's safety, would by replaced by "guards." Likewise, "patients" would be replaced by fellow "inmates."

Alternatively, one might wish to consider the use of such a paradigm in situations of "bad outcome" rather than completed suicide alone. Broadly or narrowly taken, however, the process of assessing, understanding, and developing an intervention strategy for anticipating, announcing, assisting, and assessing among family, clinicians, patients, and the associated administration can lead to improved resolution of the turmoil experienced in the aftermath of suicide.

References

Bartles SJ: The aftermath of suicide on the psychiatric inpatient unit. Gen Hosp Psychiatry 9:189–197, 1987

Bengesser G: Postvention for bereaved family members: some therapeutic possibilities. Crisis 9(1):45–48, 1988

Bolton I: My Son–My Son: A Guide to Healing After Death, Loss, or Suicide. Atlanta, Bolton Press, 1983

Chance S: Surviving suicide: a journey to resolution. Bull Menninger Clin 52:30–39, 1988

Cooper C: Psychiatric stress debriefing: alleviating the impact of patient suicide and assault. J Psychosoc Nurs Ment Health Serv 33:21–25, 1995

Cotton PG, Drake RE Jr, Whitaker A, et al: Dealing with suicide on a psychiatric inpatient unit. Hospital and Community Psychiatry 34:55–59, 1983

Dunne-Maxim K, Godin S, Lamb F, et al: The aftermath of youth suicide—providing postvention services for the school and community. Crisis 13(1):16–22, 1992

Fawcett J, Clark DC, Busch KA: Assessing and treating the patient at risk for suicide. Psychiatric Annals 23:244–255, 1993

Fine C: No Time to Say Goodbye: Surviving the Suicide of a Loved One. New York, Doubleday, 1997

Hewett JH: After Suicide. Louisville, KY, Westminster John Knox Press, 1980
Hodgkinson PE: Responding to inpatient suicide. Br J Med Psychol 60:387–392, 1987
Kaye NS, Soreff SM: The psychiatrist's role, responses, and responsibilities when a patient commits suicide. Am J Psychiatry 148:739–743, 1991
Litman R: When patients commit suicide. Am J Psychother 19:570–576, 1965
Neill K, Benensohn HS, Farber AN, et al: The psychological autopsy: a technique for investigating a hospital suicide, Hospital and Community Psychiatry 25:33–36, 1974
Roy A: Risk factors for suicide in psychiatric patients. Arch Gen Psychiatry 39:1089–1095, 1982
Stelovich S: Framework for handling adverse events. Forum (Risk Management Foundation of the Harvard Medical Institutions), April 1997, pp 8–9
Webster's Seventh New Collegiate Dictionary. Springfield, MA, G & C Merriam Company, 1963

APPENDIX A

The Formulation of Suicide Risk

John T. Maltsberger, M.D.

The "formulation of suicide risk" is a disciplined method for assessing suicide danger. It integrates and balances the presenting clinical material from the patient's past history, his present illness, and the present mental state examination. There are five components in case formulation: 1) assessing the patient's past responses to stress, especially losses; 2) assessing the patient's vulnerability to three life-threatening affects—aloneness, self-contempt, and murderous rage; 3) determining the nature, availability, and utility of exterior sustaining resources; 4) assessing the emergence and emotional importance of death fantasies; and 5) assessing the patient's capacity for reality testing.

With practice the necessary interviewing and data organizing can be accomplished in about an hour's time. The *history of the present illness* is obtained first, the *mental state* is examined, *pertinent past and family history* are reviewed, and then the findings are organized.

In taking the history the examiner should bear in mind the following common correlates of suicide completion:

This appendix was condensed and modified from Maltsberger JT: "Suicide Danger: Clinical Estimation and Decision." *Suicide and Life-Threatening Behavior* 18:47–54, 1988.

- Axis I disorders: depression, alcoholism, drug abuse, schizophrenia
- Recent suicidal behavior: attempts, preparations, plans, communications to others
- Prior suicide attempts, especially those of high lethality
- Isolation: living alone, divorce, death, emotional abandonment by significant others
- Recent loss
- Mental anguish: "psychache," self-hate, and hopelessness
- Elderly white male
- Family history of or identification with a suicide completer
- Economic reverses
- Physical illness
- Combinations of any of the above (raises risk)

Past Responses to Stress

The patient's past responses to stress come to light through study of his past history. Particular attention should be paid to such moments of challenge as going off to school; adolescent development; disappointments in love, work, or academic life; family strains; deaths of relatives, friends, children, or pets; divorce; and such other hurts and losses as may be discovered. Here the examiner tries to discern and get a grip on consistent lifelong coping patterns. We assume that patients will tend to cope in the future as they have coped in the past.

A man who responded to the death of his mother 10 years ago with a depression from which he recovered after some psychotherapy can probably survive the death of a best friend without becoming suicidal if the positive resources in his psychological field remain unchanged. But if at his mother's death the patient withdrew from others, overdosed, developed an alcohol problem, or manifested a psychosis, there may be trouble in store. Of special interest in assessing coping patterns will be any history of previous suicide attempts and their nature, purposes, and gravity. In addition, the examiner will want to know on whom or on what the patient has relied to keep going in troubled times. The examiner will also want to know whether the patient has been vulnerable to depression in the past, and whether he has been prone to abandon hope in the face of trouble—in other words, whether the patient is vulnerable to despair. Despair is much more highly correlated with suicide and serious suicide attempts than is depression.

Vulnerability to Life-Threatening Affects

The central stimulus to most suicides is intolerable psychic pain (Shneidman 1993). Patients who reach maturity with serious difficulty in emotional self-regulation are at risk to be overwhelmed with emotional agony unless there is some outside supportive intervention.

The first variety of potentially lethal pain is *aloneness*, the subjective correlate of utter emotional abandonment. Aloneness is different from lonesomeness. Lonesomeness is an experience softened with hope, experienced as limited in time, eased by memories of love and closeness, and attenuated with the expectation of closeness to come again. Aloneness is, however, in its most extreme form, an experience devoid of hope. In the full flood of aloneness, the patient feels that there has never been love, that there will never be love, and that he is dying. This is the anxiety of annihilation—an evil amalgam of panic and terror. People will do anything to escape from this experience. The frantic patient in an agitated depression who plucks at the clothes of passers-by, begging for relief, experiences something of aloneness. Edvard Munch's famous picture "The Scream" evokes a slight echo of aloneness in many of us. Many patients with anxiety disorders and borderline personality disorders are vulnerable to aloneness.

The second variety of killing psychic pain is *self-contempt*. Self-contempt in the patient close to suicide is different from ordinary anger at oneself not only quantitatively but qualitatively as well. To be sure, the patient may be deeply and scornfully self-contemptuous. The subjective experience is not only uncomfortable; it is an interior scalding. Qualitatively, it differs also from low self-esteem, because these patients feel subjectively separate from their hating consciences. One patient said he felt that he was trapped in his body at the mercy of a torturer.

Distinct from self-hate but akin to it is the incapacity for self-appreciation. Those with this incapacity feel worthless, valueless, and unlovable. It is easier for people to bear the heat of a burning conscience if they feel they have some merit, in spite of all. Those who feel valueless have much greater difficulty standing up against an interior attack because they do not believe they are worth saving.

The third variety of dangerous psychic pain is *murderous rage*. Patients may bear ordinary anger, but when murderous hate holds sway, patients are in danger of turning it against themselves, sometimes because their consciences will not tolerate such a feeling without passing a death sentence, but occasionally because they are protecting the lives of other people. Such patients feel their control weakening; fearing they can no longer restrain themselves from murder, they commit suicide instead.

Exterior Sustaining Resources

It is only by relying on exterior sustaining resources that those vulnerable to suicide can protect themselves from flooding by deadly affects. Unable to regulate themselves without relying on someone or something outside the core of the self, such patients nevertheless may remain in good equilibrium as long as the necessary resource is consistently and dependably available. It is the loss of the stabilizing exterior resource that is likely to precipitate an affective flood and invite suicide. The past history will commonly give good indications of what kind of resource the individual patient must have in order to maintain emotional homeostasis. There are three classes of exterior sustaining resources on which patients depend to keep in balance: others, work, and special self-aspects.

Most commonly, suicide-vulnerable people depend on *others* to feel real, to feel separate, to keep reasonably calm, and to feel reasonably valuable. The loss or threatened loss of such a sustaining other can lead to an explosion of aloneness, self-contempt, and murderous fury. Suicide is often triggered by the loss of a parent, a spouse, or a special friend. Sometimes suicide is precipitated by the death of a beloved pet. One patient has warded off suicide all her life by the companionship of a series of cats; she insists that all these cats, by now six or seven of them, are really the same original cat of her childhood. They may look slightly different on the outside, but inside each successive cat the spirit of the original lives on. This cat, by continuous transmigration of its soul, remains constant, always loving her, soothing her, valuing her, and keeping her in balance.

Sometimes patients depend not on others for maintaining equilibrium, but on their *work* instead. I recall one man raised in an emotionally aloof, somewhat cruel, cold family. Early in his schooling he developed a passion for learning. He was an extraordinarily gifted boy and rapidly progressed through elementary grades, high school, university, and graduate study with highest honors. But he remained emotionally isolated: his personal life was always a shambles; others mattered little to him except as conveniences for the meeting of physical needs. His wife said she felt like a ham sandwich. But academically he rose rapidly and precociously became an eminent professor. Learning and teaching were everything to him. It was not surprising that his retirement precipitated a suicide crisis—a crisis that was resolved only when space was made in a colleague's laboratory for some continuing research and provision was made for the teaching of a graduate seminar.

A third class of sustaining resources is *valued self-aspects*. Some part or function of the patient's own body is commonly taken as such a self-aspect; the patient experiences it as not being quite connected to the rest of his devalued self. One patient, a socially isolated accountant, paranoid and chronically suicidal, was able to live on only because of his passion for jogging. At the end of his daily run he would shower and then stand before a full-length mirror, lost in admiration of what he beheld there—a fine athletic body, the final destruction of which was unthinkable. We may refer to this patient's body as an exterior sustaining resource, because emotionally what he saw in the mirror was not experienced as a part of his central self. Neither did he experience it as quite belonging to the outside. It was for him a transitional object, and a life-sustaining one.

In this aspect of case formulation, it is important not only to identify which of the necessary sustaining resources has failed or threatens to fail, but to assess as well whether or not some important person may not actually wish the patient to be dead. Often enough after suicide has taken place, we find evidence that a relative has ignored suicide threats or otherwise complied in a patient's death through inaction.

The identification of whom or what the patient must have in order to carry on, and the determination of whether that resource is available, threatened, temporarily unavailable, or hopelessly lost, are crucial steps in the formulation of suicide risk. It is the availability of exterior resources that protects the patient from despair. *But equally important is the question of whether or not the patient can appreciate, take hold of, and use resources to keep alive.* Some patients may be so overwhelmed with pain that they abandon their attachments in the real world and can only think of taking flight. Helping hands may be held out, but the helping hands may not be grasped.

Death Fantasies: Their Presence and Emotional Valence

Assessment of the emergence and emotional importance of death fantasies is the fourth part of formulation in suicide. Though some would disagree, I believe, at least to the unconscious, there is no cessation in death. The close clinical observer usually will find that patients speaking of "putting an end to it all" really wish for something like a deep sleep, a sleep of peace. Of course sleep is not death, but for millennia people have tended to equate the two. To the unconscious, the egression of death often amounts to an emigration to another land where things will be better. Does not the word "egression" connote a going somewhere? going out? We may ask, going out to where?

Fantasies of going somewhere, joining somebody, perhaps in another life beyond the grave, need to be asked for, explored, and, when found, assessed. When fantasies of this nature are in fact delusional, or when they operate with delusional force, the patient may be in danger of suicide. In situations of intense distress, illusions may be so overvalued that they operate with the intensity of delusions. The following case illustrates this point.

> Mr. G., a 63-year-old retired office worker, was transferred to a psychiatric inpatient unit after surviving an almost lethal overdose of digitalis. A former alcoholic, the patient had overcome his difficulties and become widely known for his volunteer work. A stroke left him with a thalamic infarction. He experienced great difficulty in urinating. Frequent catheterization became necessary, and his leg brace was commonly wet with urine. The stroke also left him subject to severe attacks of pain in which his hand, arm, and leg felt as though they were being crushed in a vise or pierced with sharp needles—the worst experiences of pain in his entire life. Furthermore, his ailments forced him out of the home he had shared for some years with friends. What he ostensibly found intolerable were physical decay and the suffering for which he could find no relief. He had hoarded digitalis, planning to commit suicide for months, promising himself "escape" when the suffering became too much. But careful examination showed that in fact what made life intolerable was the loss of his dog, Fidel.
>
> When asked what he had imagined it would be like to be dead, Mr. G. began to cry and confided that he had hoped Fidel would be there "on the other side" waiting for him. He was careful to point out he had no sense of certainty, but a strong hope, about life beyond the grave. The patient told the examiner about Fidel eagerly, in great detail, weeping all the while as he explained how inseparable they had been. Fidel had accompanied him to banquets, had appeared on the platform with him, had attracted the notice of celebrities. For years, Mr. G. had secretly smuggled Fidel into movies. The dog's intelligence had been noted by everyone; the patient and his pet had enjoyed a complete mutual capacity to understand each other's thoughts and feelings. They were the closest of friends.
>
> When Fidel was 13 years old, he developed diabetes and required insulin injections; urinary incontinence followed. On the advice of the veterinarian, the dog was given "euthanasia." After cremation, his ashes were dispersed on a beach where "by coincidence" those of a friend's wife had been scattered before. Mr. G. liked to imagine Fidel frisking along beside her, keeping her company. Before this hospital admission, the patient had not seen the connection between Fidel's illness and "euthanasia" and his own incontinence and suicide attempt.

Mr. G.'s mother had been physically and emotionally abusive; he had relied on his father and brother to raise him. From the age of 14, he was never without a dog, and before that he would leave for school a half hour early in order to "have conversations with four dogs who lived in the neighborhood." When asked if he would have attempted suicide had Fidel remained at his side, Mr. G. exclaimed indignantly, "What? Leave Fidel? Never!"

Capacity for Reality Testing

Assessment of the patient's capacity for reality testing is the final aspect of the formulation of suicide danger. The foregoing example shows that in a patient caught up in despair—in this instance, the despair of aloneness—fantasies about a better life after death may operate with perilous intensity. It is important not only to inquire about such fantasies or beliefs but to decide how much psychological distance the patient can place between them and himself.

Patients in profoundly depressed states may not be able to form realistic appraisals of how much they are loved and valued by others. One must ask not only whether the external sustaining resources are available but whether the patient is able to understand and grasp that fact.

Paranoid patients may also suffer from such disturbances of reality testing that they have grown convinced others who love them are in fact dangerous traitors who want to do them ill, so that correct appreciation of the availability of others is impossible.

Conclusion

The formulative approach to assessing suicide risk outlined here (see Maltsberger 1986 for a fuller development of this approach) affords a disciplined method for weighing the various vulnerabilities and strengths of patients who threaten to destroy themselves. It also provides a means of assessing and integrating the influences, both interior and exterior, that hold such patients back from or drive them toward self-destruction.

Suggested Readings

Buie DH, Adler G: Definitive treatment of the borderline patient. Int J Psychoanal Psychother 9:51–87, 1982

Maltsberger JT: Suicide Risk: The Formulation of Clinical Judgment. New York, New York University Press, 1986

Shneidman ES: Definition of Suicide. New York, Wiley, 1985

Shneidman ES: Suicide as psychache. J Nerv Ment Dis 181:147–149, 1993

APPENDIX B

Getting More of What Is Needed From Your Patient's Managed Care Organization

James M. Ellison, M.D., M.P.H.

In this appendix, I suggest 10 tips to ease the clinician's interactions with managed care. Much of the advice included here has been covered in more detail in the preceding chapters. It is encapsulated here for review and easy reference. While I and my colleagues have found these suggestions helpful, they may not be sufficient to obtain satisfactory responses from all reviewers or with every managed care plan. Clinicians and patients may be able to obtain increased services by means of these tips but also must keep in mind that even the most generous insurance plan (and any managed care plan) is ultimately a limited source of payment that supports only treatments defined as medically necessary.

1. Know your patient's insurance benefits.

Familiarize yourself with your patient's insurance benefits at the beginning of treatment, not after authorized services are exhausted and your patient is in crisis. Be sure to obtain your patient's proper identifying information, including birth date, plan number, subscriber name, and correct address. Your patient should have received a description of benefits at the time of enrollment in the plan; if not, you can request information on benefits from the insurer. If you are a "risk averse" clinician, you may prefer to limit your practice to patients whose insurance benefits are in your opinion adequate for the services they will need. To avoid providing services that will be unreimbursed, plan ahead and know how many more sessions that patient can attend before a request for further services must be submitted.

2. Discuss coverage issues with your patient up front.

Many patients do not understand how outpatient mental health services are covered under managed care. They may believe that whatever services they "need" will be provided without understanding the limitations on coverage or the definition of "need" used by the managed care organization (MCO). In reality, even the coverage of "up to 60 inpatient days" and "up to 20 outpatient visits" per year does not guarantee that the patient will receive these benefits if the relevant diagnosis or treatment objectives are not considered by a reviewer to be "medically necessary." You and your patient will be displeased to learn of benefit limitations in the midst of a crisis. To the extent that is appropriate with your patient and remaining mindful of the patient's level of distress, therefore, discuss what will and what will not be covered up front. This discussion should include the number of outpatient sessions or inpatient days that will be initially authorized, the copayments that will be required, the procedure for obtaining further services and whatever expenses this will confer on the patient (such as a greater copayment per session for outpatient sessions after those initially approved), the name of a designated inpatient facility if the patient's options will be determined in this way, and the nature of any conditions (such as attention-deficit disorder in some plans) for which mental health services will not be readily covered through mental health benefits.

3. Discuss alternative sources of payment.

Many patients do not understand the nature of insurance, which is a financial program by which an individual contributes a fixed, regular payment in exchange for assurance of a limitation on loss due to unexpectedly large but necessary expenditures. Insurance is not meant to cover prolonged elective treatment such as an inpatient stay that is extended while suitable housing is located for an already stabilized patient or outpatient psychotherapy that the patient finds engaging and useful but is not "medically" required. Clinicians, too, may fall prey to a sense of "entitlement" regarding the limitations of insurance rather than recognizing that some services will require other sources of support. Some patients will be able to finance their extended treatment through self-payment or with help from a relative, while others may require the clinician to "slide" the fee down accordingly. Many institutions have a "free care" policy that will determine whether a patient's coverage and income entitle him or her to continued treatment at a low rate or at no cost.

4. Know the procedure for obtaining more covered services.

The patient's insurance card will most likely include a toll-free number for obtaining information about mental health benefits and/or for preauthorizing inpatient admissions. To obtain further outpatient sessions after the number initially allocated, you will probably have to fill out an "OTR," or outpatient treatment review. Although efforts are under way to standardize the information that can be requested, MCOs currently use proprietary forms for this purpose that vary greatly. If you do not provide the required information, do not be surprised to see your request returned to you, often after a substantial delay, for completion.

5. You will obtain more services with sound clinical reasoning than with threats!

Remember that the "reviewer" very likely was once (and maybe still is) a "clinician." Many reviewers work only part-time for the MCO and see patients in their other time. While urged to avoid authorization of unnecessary services, perhaps on the basis of proprietary MCO definitions of medical necessity, diagnostic criteria, and "appropriate" levels of care, these reviewers have also almost certainly been instructed to approve (within prearranged benefit limitations) care that is appropriate. Sound clinical reasoning remains the most reliable approach for obtaining the maximum services available under your patient's inpatient or outpatient mental health benefits. Understand what your patient's plan means by "medically necessary" so that you can use this language in your discussion with a reviewer. Document and discuss specific, recent changes in behavior, and be prepared to discuss how your treatment plan has helped and will continue to help. When you feel that you are speaking with a reviewer who lacks the clinical training to understand your reasoning or your patient's needs, do not hesitate to ask for the reviewer's qualifications. If necessary, ask to speak with a "clinician," and if a clinician with appropriate training (e.g., a child psychiatrist trained in pharmacotherapy in the case of a request for more child psychopharmacology services) is unavailable, be prepared to begin an appeals process if the requested services are not approved.

6. There is also a time and place for threats.

Losing your temper with a reviewer is generally an unhelpful gambit, but there are occasions when it is appropriate to remind the reviewer of the potential for adverse consequences if services are not provided. I like to start by appealing to the reviewer's clinical judgment, but when a reviewer seems unresponsive to needs that appear pressing to me (e.g., urging discharge of an inpatient who appears still quite suicidal), I change the discussion to one of "customer satisfaction." Because many MCOs are struggling to attract and enroll more members in a very competitive market, this approach may prevail. If not, my next (and most assertive) stance assures that the reviewer understands that he or she would be likely to incur corporate responsibility in the event of an adverse outcome. I ask for the reviewer's name, for the purpose of documenting this in the patient's medical record, and remind the reviewer that courts are increasingly considering MCOs to bear a *duty* to patients that such a denial of care may abrogate. Citing *Wilson v. Blue Cross of Southern California* (1990) (see Chapter 8, this volume) and current legislative efforts to remove the ERISA (Employee Retirement Income Security Act of 1974) protection of MCOs, I remind the reviewer that I have personally assessed this clinical situation and will be certain to follow through with a complaint to the insurance commissioner about what I consider an improper practice.

7. Do not hesitate to appeal when necessary services are denied.

As emphasized particularly in Chapter 8 of this book, the denial of coverage in no way absolves the treating clinician from providing appropriate care. In fact, clinicians bear liability for failing to oppose an inappropriate limitation of services, as demonstrated in the case of *Wickline v. State* (1986), a lawsuit that concluded that a physician bore responsibility for medical damage (loss of a leg) to a patient following a failure to appeal an MCO's denial of extra hospital days for the continuation of necessary postoperative care. Furthermore, denial and subsequent use of the appeal process may be a necessary step if the patient is later to seek legal redress from the MCO for inappropriate limitation of services.

8. When appropriate specialized services are not available under the plan's benefit package, advocate for their coverage.

As noted in Chapter 2 of this book, in which this issue is discussed in relation to obtaining dialectical behavior therapy services, it is sometimes possible to obtain noncovered services when there is clinical justification that makes such services "medically necessary." The clinician should initially approach this goal by demonstrating to the insurer that the requested treatment modality is known to be effective for the condition to be treated, that the failure to treat the condition in question will likely result in harm to the patient, and that utilization of the requested treatment is likely to produce a cost-saving offset by making more expensive other services less likely to be required. With advocacy of this sort, it may be possible to obtain authorization for various specialty consultations, laboratory procedures, nonformulary medications, and other exceptional interventions for which coverage would otherwise be denied.

9. Keep an open mind during review discussions.

It is worth bearing in mind that the MCO is not inherently an "evil" force, even though its attention to cost-effectiveness makes it unfamiliar and suspect to many clinicians. As emphasized throughout this book, the MCO may have unique and valuable services to offer a patient by virtue of containing or contracting with a network of services that are of varying levels of intensity. When your request to the MCO for a patient's continued treatment meets with refusal, ask what other options are available to the patient.

10. Remember to take your own pulse.

When feelings of frustration and anger arise during discussions with MCOs, keep in mind that the success and spread of managed care represents a societal choice even though it may impose some barriers to clinical services. Indeed, it is possible that you yourself have chosen the less costly premiums associated with a managed care product rather than purchase a more expensive insurance. Many of our patients have not had the option to choose otherwise, since their employers may offer a very limited selection of insurances or their incomes may limit their choices. We must avoid taking out our frustration on them or turning the anger inward. Usually a solution can be found!

INDEX

Page numbers printed in **boldface** *type refer to tables or figures.*

Abandonment, alcoholics' feeling of, 4–5
Abille v. United States, 159
Access to care, 16
   designated central screening facility for, 120
   as inadvertent reinforcer of suicidal behavior, 33
   in managed crisis care, 23–24, 27
   triage in managed system and problems of, 42–43
Accidental poisoning, alcohol abuse and, 5
Acute event, distinguishing between chronic behaviors and, 82. *See also* Chronically suicidal patient
Acutely suicidal patient, effective managed care of
   assessment, 29
   longer-term care, 30
Acute residential treatment, 53–55
Administrators. *See* Authorities, aftermath of suicide and
Admission. *See also* Inpatient setting/care
   calling managed care system to request, 34
   commitment criteria, 45
Adolescents in managed care, suicidal, 59–84
   acute residential care, 53
   chain of appeals for, 75–77
   drug rehabilitation for, 68
   dual diagnosis creep and, 68–70
   evaluating, 60–64
   evolving treatment models for, 64–65
   excluded conditions and treatments, 73–74
   family treatment for, 75
   geographic cures, 71–72
   medical necessity with, 72–73
   medication vs. talking cures for, 70–71
   new responsibilities regarding, 77–78
   rate of suicide among, 59–60, 77
   responsible care of, 65–68
   speeding patient assessment, 62–64
   substance abuse and, 60–61, 112
   tips for treating, 80–84
Advocacy for services
   additional care, 43
   for the elderly, tips for, 98, **99**
   specialized services, 201
Affects, vulnerability to life-threatening, 191–192
Aftermath of suicide, needs and interventions in, 173–187
   announcing, **177**, 180–181
   anticipating, **177**, 178–180
   assessing, **177**, 184–185
   assisting, **177**, 181–184
   groups affected, 174–177
Agency for Health Care Policy and Research, "Depression in Primary Care" clinical practice guidelines of, 97

Agitation, crisis assessment and
symptom of, 18
Akathisia, 137
Alcohol use/abuse, 4–5
crisis assessment and symptom of, 18
pharmacotherapy for, 135
suicidality and, 111, 112, 113
Algorithms
for effective assessment, 28–29
for utilization management and
clinical decision-making, 26
Alienation, 46
Aloneness, 191
Alprazolam, 136
American Association of Suicidology
(AAS), 95
American College of
Neuropsychopharmacology, 137
American Foundation for Suicide
Prevention, 174
Amitriptyline, 136, 139
Anabolic steroids, 137
Anguish, 2–3
Announcing suicide of patient, 177,
180–181
Anticholinergic tricyclics, 144
Anticipatory component of treatment,
177, 178–180
Antidepressants
inadequate dosage of, 92, 93
overdose with, 138–139
prescribed by primary care
clinicians, 139–140
selective serotonin reuptake
inhibitor (SSRI), 93
serotonergic, 133–134
serotonin reuptake inhibitor, 93,
138, 144–145
treatment-emergent suicidality
associated with, 135–137
tricyclic, 139, 144
Antisocial personality disorder, alcohol
use and, 113

Anxiety
depressive disorder and, 3, 4
of partial hospital clinician, 50
Anxiety disorders, suicidal behavior
and, 118–119
Appeal boards, independent managed
care, 169
Appeals
chain of, for adolescents, 75–77
of denials of medical treatments, 74,
83–84
for necessary services, 200–201
process of, following, 168
Appointments, pharmacotherapy
follow-up on missed, 146
frequency and length of, based on
patient needs, 141–142
Assessing meaning of suicide, 177,
184–185
Assessment
acute, for suicidal substance abusers
in managed care, 116–120
for brief hospitalization, 48
in crisis care, 16–19
managed crisis care, 24–25,
27–28
elements of adequate, 158
expedited, 62–64
formulation of suicide risk,
189–196
capacity for reality testing, 195
death fantasies, 193–195
exterior sustaining resources,
192–193
past responses to stress in, 190
vulnerability to life-threatening
affects, 191–192
lessons learned from cases
involving, 160
professional judgment and, 158
of suicidality, 45, 47
Assisting affected groups coping with
suicide, 177, 181–184

Index

Authorities, aftermath of suicide and, 175–176, **177**
  announcing suicide of patient to, 180–181
  anticipatory component of treatment and, 178
  assessing meaning of suicide and, 184
  assistance for, to cope with suicide, 181, 182–183
Auxiliary informants. *See* Collateral informants, gathering data from
Availability of services, 23

"Baby boomers," suicide rates among, 87
Barriers to care, managed care access experienced as, 23–24. *See also* Access to care
Beck Hopelessness Scale, 17, 28
Behavioral analysis in dialectical behavior therapy, 31–32
Behavioral managed care programs, 77
Behavior therapy, procedure for seeking approval for course of, 70–71
Bellah v. Greenson, 157, 161
Bell v. New York City Health & Hospitals Corp., 158
Benefits, flexible options for use of, 68, 123
Benzodiazepines
  for depression in the elderly, 93
  suicide attempts by women using, 112
  suicide by overdose of, 138
  unpleasant discontinuation syndrome associated with, 144–145
Biological markers of suicidal behavior, 88–89

Bipolar mood disorders, lithium treatment for, 133
Blood tests to assess acutely suicidal substance abuser, 117
Borderline personality disorder
  dialectical behavior therapy for chronically suicidal patient with, 30–32
  pharmacotherapy for, 136
  reduction in suicidal ideation/behavior and, 134
Brandt v. Grubin, 161
Brandvain v. Ridgeview Institute, Inc., 159
Breach of trust, suicide attempt signifying patient's experience of, 21
Brief hospitalization, 48–50

Cancer, risk of suicide in elderly with, 90
Capacity for reality testing, 195
Capitation rates, 164–166, 167
Carbamazepine, 134
Care, duty of, 154
Case management, 123–124
  compliance improved by, 126
Case manager
  establishing working relationship with, 34
  monitoring of, 63–64
  negotiating with, 35
Case-rated hospitals, 67
Causation, 164
Central Anesthesia Associates, P.C. v. Worthy, 156n
Cerebrospinal fluid (CSF) 5-hydroxyindoleacetic acid (5-HIAA), 88–89
Change, addressing patient's needs in maintaining, 49
Children in acute residential care, 53. *See also* Adolescents in managed care, suicidal

Chronically suicidal patient, 18–19
    advantage of managed care for, 26
    assessment, 29
    longer-term care, 30–31
    increased outpatient supports for, 43–44
    triggering stimulus for, identifying, 46
"Chronic care" benefit, 125
Clinical decision-making, guidelines or algorithms for, 26
Clinical guidelines
    development of, in managed care system, 26–27
    for managed crisis care, 34–36
    for working with suicidal substance abusers, **127–128**
Clinician(s)
    aftermath of suicide and, 175, **177**
        announcing suicide of patient, 180–181
        anticipatory component of treatment and, 178
        assessing meaning of suicide, 184
        assistance for, to cope with suicide, 181–182
    assessment of own responses to patient, 17–18
    changing, 10, 76
    duties of. *See* Duty, clinician's
    emergency room, communicating with, 41, 43
    inpatient, constraints on, 48, 49
    interactions with managed care, tips for, 197–202
    outpatient
        as advocate for additional care, 43
        longer-term risk of suicide as work of, 46
        partial hospital, 50–51
        previous therapist, gathering data from, 81
        primary care. *See* Primary care physicians
Clozapine, 134
CNA HealthPro, 156
Cocaine use, suicide risk and, 112, 113
Cognitive-behavioral approach
    for chronically suicidal patient, 30–31
    to crisis intervention, 20
Cohen v. State of New York, 158
Collaboration, managed care hospital, 66–67
Collateral informants, gathering data from, 43. *See also* Family
    assessing acutely suicidal substance abuser and, 117
    reassessment and, 121
    for suicidal adolescent, 81
College students, treating, 71–72
Command hallucinations, deadly augury of, 6
Commitment criteria, 45
Communication
    between clinicians in managed care system, 24
    with emergency room clinicians, 41, 43
    miscommunication, 11
    with ongoing treaters, 21
    oral, with team members, 160
    of suicidal intent, 93
Community psychiatry movement, 67
Comorbidity, crisis assessment and presence of, 18
Compensation, treatment decision determined by, 164–169. *See also* Insurance coverage
Confidentiality, 117, 121, 159, 161–162
Consultation
    crisis assessment as, 21

Index

defense of later allegation of negligence and, 161
in managed care, 23
when to initiate psychiatric, 99
"Contagion" phenomenon, 62
Contingency management, 33–34
Contingency plans, 19
"Continuous care" spectrum, 40, 123
acute residential treatment, 53–55
brief hospitalization, 48–50
focal treatment planning, 44–48
observation/holding beds, 55–56, 121–122
partial hospitalization, 50–53, 67, 68
triage in managed system, 41–44
triage-oriented formulation and, 44–48
Contract(s)
dialectical behavior therapy, 33–34
"no-harm," emergency use of, 19
reliance on, 8–9
Contract negotiations, provider/managed care, 167
Contractual termination clauses, 168–169
Coordination of care
following discharge from partial hospital program, 50
from outpatient providers, 123
standards of care, 29
Coping skills, sobriety and need for, 126
Coping strategies, 19
consistent lifelong coping patterns, 190
constructing personalized list of, 33
Corcoran v. United HealthCare, 166
Corporate employees, narrow treatment focus with, 72–73
Cost-containment, 26, 164–166
Costs of acute residential vs. inpatient care, 54

Counseling, as immediate intervention, 20
Couples therapy dedicated to issues concerning child, 75
Crisis, as time of danger and opportunity, 16
Crisis care, 16–22
access, 16
assessment, 16–19
immediate intervention, 19–20
innovative programs for the elderly, 96–97
longer-term care, laying groundwork for, 20–22
in managed care. *See* Managed crisis care
Crisis prevention centers, elderly use of, 95–96
Crisis survival strategies, 32
Cross-discipline reporting relationships, 163
Customer satisfaction, appealing to reviewer by discussing, 200
Cycling affective illness, 18

Dangerousness, assessment of, 17–18, 116
DBT. *See* Dialectical behavior therapy (DBT)
Death fantasies, 193–195
Decision making
duty to exercise proper judgment in, 157–161
guidelines or algorithms for clinical, 26
treatment decisions, insurance coverage and, 160–161, 164–169
Delusions, 6, 194
Demographic risk factors
crisis assessment and, 18
for the elderly, 98

Depression, 56
    age-related variations in diagnosis
        and treatment of, 93
    alcohol use and, 4–5, 113
    in the elderly, suicide and, 85,
        91–92
    electroconvulsive treatment for,
        reluctance to prescribe, 9–10
    mental health care delivery for,
        85–86, 92–95
    payment plan and detection rate of
        unipolar, 93–94
    pharmacotherapy for. See also
        Antidepressants
        reduction in suicidal ideation/
            behavior with, 133–134
        slow response to, 9
    psychotic, overlooking suicidal
        shifts in patients recovering
        from, 8
    in schizophrenic patients, 5–6
    substance abuse to relieve, 118–119
Depression questionnaires, 98
Designated facility
    advantage/disadvantage to using,
        52–53
    for screening, 120
Desipramine, 139
Despair, vulnerability to, 190
Detoxification, 20
Diagnosis, 2–6
    of alcoholism, 4–5
    crisis assessment and, 17
    of depressive illness, 2–4
    dual diagnosis creep, 68–70
    duty to exercise proper judgment in,
        157–161
    of psychoses, 5–6
Dialectical behavior therapy (DBT),
    30–36
    behavioral analysis in, 31–32
    clinical guidelines for, 35–36
    treatment contract, 33–34

Diazepam, 137
Discharge. See also Levels of care
    failure to reexamine patient before,
        7–8
    overlooking suicidal shifts in
        recovering patients after, 8
    premature, 63, 64
Discipline-specific level of reasonable
    care, 154
Disclosure to policyholder about
    treatment of dependent, 75
Discontinuation of drugs, avoiding
    abrupt, 144–145
Discontinuity of care, 10
Disease management model, case
    management using, 123–124
Disposition
    immediate intervention and, 20
    treatment protocols in managed care
        systems, 121
Disposition plan
    for brief hospitalization, 48
    development of, 30
    use of observation beds and, 55–56
Distress tolerance skills, 32
Disulfiram, 135
Documentation. See also Medical
    records
    of assessment, 160
    duty to document, 158–159
    of risk-benefit analysis of clinical
        decisions, 160, 168
    of suicidality, 45, 47
Dothiepin, 139
Drug rehabilitation, 68, 69–70,
    124–125
Dual diagnosis creep, 68–70
Duty, clinician's, 156–163
    duty of care, 154
    duty to exercise proper judgment in
        diagnosis and treatment
        decisions, 157–161
    duty to protect, 157

Index

duty to supervise, 162–163
duty to warn/duty to maintain patients' confidentiality, 161–162
Dysphoric Affect Scale, 3, 4

Education program on elderly depression and suicide, 100
Effectiveness of treatment, demonstrating, 82
Elderly, suicide in, 85–110
   advocating for managed care services, tips for, 98, **99**
   biology of, 88–89
   demographic factors correlated with increased, 98
   epidemiology of, 86–88
   gender differences and, 86, 89, 92
   physical illness and, 89–90, 91
   premises of managed care organizations addressing, 101
   prevention of, 95–102
     primary prevention efforts, 101
     secondary prevention efforts, 101–102
     tertiary prevention strategies, 102
   primary care physician and, 85–86, 92–93, 97–98
   psychopathology of, 90–95
Electroconvulsive therapy (ECT), 9–10, 134
Emergency psychiatric services, 28
Emergency room services
   access in managed care to, 24
   crisis assessment, 17
   elderly use of, 97–98
   immediate transport for, 20
Emergency triage protocols, 41–44
Employee benefits office, appeal to, 76
Epidemiology of suicide in elderly, 86–88

ERISA (Employee Retirement Income Security Act of 1974)
   preemptions, 166–167, 200
Evaluations. *See* Assessment
Excluded conditions and treatments, 73–74
Expectations of care
   in crisis management, 21
   marketing of managed care and unrealistic, 120
Exterior sustaining resources, 192–193
"Extracontractual benefits," request for providing, 76–77

Face-to-face evaluation, 19
Failure to monitor resulting in suicide, 156
Failure to prevent suicide and/or homicide, 156
Family. *See also* Collateral informants, gathering data from
   aftermath of suicide and, 174–175, 177
   announcing suicide of patient to, 180–181
   anticipatory component of treatment and, 178
   assessing meaning of suicide, 184
   assistance for, to cope with suicide, 181, 182
   documenting comments and concerns of, 160
   suicidal adolescent evaluation and, 61
Family evaluation, 19
Family therapy, 71
Family treatment, for suicidal adolescents, 75
Fantasies
   death, 193–195
   of suicide attempters, 61
Farwell v. Un, 157

Fee, provider/patient relationship and duty with or without, 156–157
Fee-for-service plan, managed system compared with, 25n, 26
  health outcomes for elderly and poor, 94
Flexible options for use of benefits, 68, 123
Fluoxetine, 133–134, 136–137
Flupentixol, 134
Fluvoxamine, 133–134
Focal treatment planning, 44–48
Follow-up care
  access to, 16
  of suicidal substance abusers in managed care, 120, 122–124
Follow-up on missed appointments, 146
Foreseeability, 164
Formulation of suicide risk, 189–196
  capacity for reality testing, 195
  death fantasies, 193–195
  exterior sustaining resources, 192–193
  past responses to stress in, 190
  vulnerability to life-threatening affects, 191–192
For-profit managed system, 25n
Free care, referring patient to sources of, 168
"Free care" policy, 199

"Gag clauses," 169
Gender differences in suicide among the elderly, 86
  physical illness and, 89
  treatment and, 92
Geographic cures, 71–72
Geriatric Outreach Program (San Francisco), 96
Geriatric suicidal behavior. *See* Elderly, suicide in

Goals of suicidal behavior or ideation, 117–118
Gregory v. Robinson, 157
Group home, 66
Gun access, evaluating suicidal adolescent and, 61–62

Hallucinations, command, 6
Harm, risk of, 164
  malpractice and, 155
Harris v. Woman's Hospital, 165
Harvard Medical Practice Study, 156
Helling v. Carey, 154
Heroin use, suicidal behavior and, 113, 135
"High lethality," determining, 26–27
History taking, 189–190. *See also* Information gathering
  inadequate, 6–7
HMO (health maintenance organization), 22n
Holding beds, 55–56, 121–122
Homere v. State of New York, 160
Homovanillic acid (HVA), 88–89
Hopelessness, 3, 4, 62
Horak v. Biris, 164
Hospitalization. *See also* Inpatient setting/care
  brief, 48–50
  case-rated hospitals, 67
  commitment criteria for, 45
  emergency room assessment for, 41
  "nonspecific therapeutic factors" in, 63
  observation bed usage and rate of, 55
  partial, 50–53, 67, 68
  premature discharge from, 63, 64
  risk of referral for, 40–41
  of suicide attempters, operational criteria for utilization review of, 26
  triage in managed system for, 41–44

Index

Hotlines, 16
  elderly use of, 95–96
Huntley v. State, 157
5-Hydroxyindoleacetic acid,
  cerebrospinal fluid, 88–89
Hypomanic upswing, 8

Imitation, suicide, 62
Immediate intervention in crisis care,
  19–20
  managed crisis care, 25–27, 28–29
Independent managed care appeal
  boards, 169
Independent practice association (IPA),
  22*n*
Information gathering. *See also*
  Collateral informants, gathering
  data from
  duty of, 158–160
  history taking, 6–7, 189–190
  need to respond to new information,
    160
Information systems of managed care
  organization, benefits of
  comprehensive, 115, 120
Informed consent, 169–170
Inhibition, alcohol use and, 113
Inpatient setting/care
  acute residential care compared
    with, 53–54
  admission criteria, 45
  admission to locked psychiatric
    unit, 21
  adolescents in, 64–65
  discontinuity of care in transition
    between outpatient and, 10
  duty to protect in, 157
  milieu therapy model of, 64–65
  procedure-oriented model of, 65
  reserved for high lethality patients,
    26–27
  short-term risk of suicide and,
    46

Insurance coverage
  alternative sources of payments,
    discussing, 198–199
  discussing coverage issues with
    patient, 198
  knowing procedure for obtaining
    more covered services, 199
  knowing your patient's coverage
    benefits, 197–198
  exclusions and limitations, 83
  preparing information for patients
    on, 168
  of specialized services, advocacy for,
    201
  stop-loss insurance, 168
  treatment decisions and, 160–161,
    164–169
Interferon, 137
Internet-based pharmacy business, 142
Interns, standard of care for
  psychiatric, 154
Intoxication, determining patient's type
  and degree of, 116. *See also*
  Substance abuse
IPA (independent practice association),
  22*n*
Isolation, social, 46
  alcohol use and, 113

Judgment
  alcohol use and impaired, 113
  in diagnosis and treatment
    decisions, duty to exercise
    proper, 157–161

Kaiser Permanente, lethality scale used
  to assess patients at, 29
Kerker v. Hurwitz, 160

Language of managed care
  focusing treatment report to speak,
    81
  of medical necessity, using, 35

Least restrictive levels of care, 25–26
Levels of care
  appropriate, 25, 28
  discipline-specific level of reasonable care, 154
  interrelationships between, 120
  least restrictive, 25–26
  in step-down program, 66–68, 82–83
Liability for negligence, 154–156
"Likelihood of serious harm," assessment of, 17
Lithium, 133
Lonesomeness, 191
Longer-term care, laying groundwork for, 20–22
  in managed crisis care, 27, 29–34

Mail-order pharmacy business, 142
Maintenance treatment to prevent relapse, justifying, 82
Major depression, 56, 94. *See also* Depression
Malpractice, 155–156, 176
Managed care
  basic expectation of patients in, 160
  contract negotiations, 168
  risks particular to, 164–170
    allowing compensation to determine treatment decisions, 164–169
    informed consent, 169–170
    rational risk management principles and, 140–146
  tips to ease clinician's interactions with, 197–202
  types of, 22*n*
Managed care environment, treating suicidal patients in, 1–13
  diagnosis, 2–6
    of alcoholism, 4–5
    of depressive illness, 2–4
    of psychoses, 5–6

pitfalls and snares in, 6–11
  changing clinicians, 10, 76
  failure to reexamine patient carefully, 7–8
  inadequate history taking, 6–7
  miscommunication, 11
  overlooking suicidal shifts in recovering patients, 8
  reliance on "contracts," 8–9
  reluctance to prescribe electroconvulsive treatment, 9–10
Managed crisis care, 22–27
  access, 23–24, 27
  assessment, 24–25, 27–28
  clinical guidelines for, 34–36
  effective, 27–34
  immediate intervention, 25–27, 28–29
  longer-term care, laying groundwork for, 27, 29–34
Managed entitlement plan (MEP), 22*n*
Maprotiline, 134, 135, 139
Marijuana users, suicidal behavior in, 114
Marital status, suicide among the elderly and, 87
Marital therapy, dedicated to issues concerning child, 75
McCullough v. Hutzel Hospital, 162
Media scrutiny of pharmacotherapy, 131
Medical care
  artificial separation of mental health care and, 91
  integration of mental health care and, 39–40
"Medical" exclusions, 74
Medical necessity
  advocating for specialized services as, 201
  appeal for reimbursement on basis of acute, 43
  criteria for, 65
  definitions of, 72

Index

with suicidal adolescents, 72–73
understanding patient's plan and meaning of, 199–200
using language of, 35
Medical Outcomes Study, 93–94
Medical records
  access to automated, in managed crisis care, 24
  adequate entries in, 158–159
  adequate review of, 158
  comprehensive information systems and, 115, 120
Medicare risk contract (MRC), 90
Medication. *See also* Pharmacotherapy, psychiatric
  alcohol abuse and errors in, 5
  as immediate intervention, 20
  implementing suicide with, 138–139
Mental anguish, 2–3
Mental disorders
  crisis assessment and presence of, 18
  psychiatric pharmacotherapy for, 132–135
Mental health services
  artificial separation of general medical and, 91
  elderly use of, 95–96
  expenditures on, 90
  integration of medical care and, 39–40
MEP (managed entitlement plan), 22n
Methadone maintenance, 135
Mianserin, 134
MICA (mentally ill chemically dependent), 68
Milieu therapy model of inpatient treatment, 64–65
Mindfulness, 31, 32
Miscommunication, 11
Monoamine oxidase inhibitors (MAOIs), 136–137

Mood disorders. *See also* Depression
  lithium treatment and, 133
  suicide in elderly and, 91–92
Multiaxial rating systems, 17
Multidisciplinary treatment plan, 48–49
Murderous rage, 191–192

Naltrexone, 135
National Center for Health Statistics (NCHS), 86
National Institute of Mental Health, 112
National standard of care, 156, 162–163
Negligence, 154–156
Neuroleptics, 138
"No-harm contract," emergency use of, 19
Noradrenergic reuptake inhibitors, 139
Nortriptyline, 139
Nurses in training, standard of care for, 154–155

Observation, as immediate intervention, 20
Observation/holding beds, 55–56, 121–122
Opiate abuse, 113–114, 135
Oral communication to team members, 160
Outpatient setting/care
  discontinuity of care in transition between inpatient and, 10
  duty to protect in, 157
  greater numbers of patients in, 1
  as too little care, recognizing, 40–41
  trimming services and cutting costs in, 39–40
Outpatient treatment review (OTR), 199
Overdose, prescription drug, 138–139

213

Paddock v. Chacko, 161
Pain, psychic, 191–192
Panic attacks, 3, 18
Parasuicidal behavior, 18–19, 31. *See also* Suicide attempts
Paroxetine, 133–134, 135
Partial hospitalization, 50–53, 67, 68
Past responses to stress, 190
Patient Assessment Tool, 17
Patients sharing treatment resources, aftermath of suicide and, 175, **177**
  announcing suicide of patient to, 180–181
  anticipatory component of treatment and, 178
  assessing meaning of suicide, 184
  assistance for, to cope with suicide, 181, 182
Personality disorders
  crisis assessment and presence of, 18
  hospitalization and, 21
  substance abuse with comorbid, 118
Pharmacotherapist, 44*n*
Pharmacotherapy, psychiatric, 9, 131–151
  effects of medications on suicide risk, 132–139
    increase in suicide risk, 135–137
    reduction of suicidal ideation and behavior, 132–135
    use of medications to implement suicide, 138–139
  as immediate intervention, 19–20
  psychotherapy combined with, 141–142
  psychotherapy vs., 70–71
  rational risk management principles in managed care, 140–146
    abrupt discontinuation of drugs, avoiding, 144–145
    follow-up on missed appointments, 146

least toxic effective drug, choosing, 145–146
    medications dispensed consistent with clinical needs and risks, 142–143
    pharmacotherapy appointments based on patient needs, 141–142
    refills with adequate clinical monitoring, 143–144
    undertreatment, avoidance of, 144
  risks of, in managed care system, 139–140
Phenobarbital, 137
Physical illness, suicide in elderly and, 89–90, 91
Point-of-service (POS), 22*n*
Police aid in involuntary commitment, 42
Policyholder, disclosure about treatment of dependent to, 75
Polysubstance ingestion, suicidal behavior and, 114
Precertification process, managed care, 24
Precipitants to suicide attempt, 49, 62
Preferred provider organization (PPO), 22*n*
Premature discharge, 63, 64
Prescription drug overdose, 138–139
Preventive care
  for the elderly, 95–102
  for suicidal substance abusers in managed care, 115
Primary care physicians, 43
  antidepressants prescribed by, 139–140
  assignment of elderly patients with depression to, 85–86, 92
  detection of depression, 86, 92
  improving mental health by attending to general geriatric care, 97–98

treatment of depression, 92–93
early identification of substance
abusers by, 115
Procedure-oriented model of inpatient
treatment, 65
ProMutual Group, 156
Protect, duty to, 157
Protocols
to determine appropriate
disposition, 30
for effective assessment, 28–29
emergency triage, 41–44
Provisional treatment plan for suicidal
adolescents, 80
Proximate cause, 164
Psychiatric hospital. *See*
Hospitalization; Inpatient setting/
care
Psychiatric illness. *See* Mental
disorders
Psychic pain, intolerable, 191–192
Psychodynamic factors in evaluation of
suicidal adolescent, 61
Psychological and Physical Sickness
Scales, 94
Psychotherapy
pharmacotherapy combined with,
141–142
pharmacotherapy vs., 70–71
Psychotic depressions, overlooking
suicidal shifts in patients
recovering from, 8

Race, suicide and
among adolescents, 60
among the elderly, 86–87
Rage, murderous, 191–192
Rapport in history taking, 7
Rating scales
multiaxial rating systems, 17
to support assessment, 28–29
Reacculturation, sobriety and, 126
Reality testing, capacity for, 195

Reasonable care, discipline-specific
level of, 154
Reassessment of suicidal substance
abusers in managed care, 121–122
Recidivists, goals of suicidal behavior
in, 117–118
Records. *See* Medical records
Recovering patients, overlooking
suicidal shifts in, 8
Reduced-fee care, 168
Reexamination of patient, 7–8
Referral
for hospitalization, risk of, 40–41
for longer-term care, 20–21
of substance abuser for follow-up
care, 122–124
targeting depressed elderly in crisis,
96
when to initiate, 99
Refills of medications, clinical
monitoring of, 143–144
Rehabilitation, drug, 68, 69–70,
124–125
Reinforcer, access as inadvertent,
33
Relapse, pharmacotherapy treatment
only and, 70
Relapse prevention, 68
justifying maintenance treatment
for, 82
Reliance on "contracts," 8–9
Reporting relationships, cross-
discipline(s), 163
Research on geriatric suicidal behavior,
future, 100–101
Residential drug rehabilitation
programs, 68
Residential treatment, acute, 53–55
Residents, standard of care for
psychiatric, 154
Resources
exterior sustaining, 192–193
suicide risk and limited, 119

Responsibility in large managed systems, dilution of clinical, 24–25
"Responsible care" treatment model, 65–68
Reviewer
　appealing to clinical judgment of, 200
　keeping open mind during discussions with, 201
Review process, expedited, 43
Risk-benefit analysis of clinical decisions, documenting, 160, 168
Risk factors
　demographic, crisis assessment and, 18
　evaluating, in suicidal adolescent, 81
　formulation of suicide risk, 189–196
　short-term vs. long-term risk of suicide, 46
Risk Management Foundation of the Harvard Medical Institutions, 163
Risk management issues, 153–172
　causation, 164
　clinician's duty, 156–163
　　duty to exercise proper judgment in diagnosis and treatment decisions, 157–161
　　duty to protect, 157
　　duty to supervise, 162–163
　　duty to warn/duty to maintain patients' confidentiality, 161–162
　foreseeability, 164
　harm, 164
　managed care, risks particular to, 164–170
　　allowing compensation to determine treatment decisions, 164–169
　　informed consent, 169–170
　　negligence and standard of care, 154–156
　　proximate cause, 164
Risk management principles in managed care, rational, 140–146
　abrupt discontinuation of drugs, avoiding, 144–145
　follow-up on missed appointments, 146
　least toxic effective drug, choosing, 145–146
　medications dispensed consistent with clinical needs and risks, 142–143
　pharmacotherapy appointments based on patient needs, 141–142
　refills with adequate clinical monitoring, 143–144
　undertreatment, avoidance of, 25–26, 144
Risk management strategies
　for assessment, 160
　confidentiality and, 161–162
　for provider/managed care contract negotiations, 167
　for supervisors of mental health care trainees, 163
　for treatment decisions amid cost-containment pressures, 165

St. Louis, Missouri, Life Crisis Services, Link-Plus component of, 96
San Francisco Suicide Prevention Center, Center for Elderly Suicide Prevention and Grief Related Services, 96
Schizophrenia, 5–6, 133, 134
Screening facility, designated central, 120
Screening process for depression or suicide risk, broadening scope of, 98
Sedative-hypnotics, abrupt cessation of, 144–145
Self-appreciation, incapacity for, 191

Index

Self-aspects as exterior sustaining resource, valued, 193
Self-contempt, 191
Self-hate, anguish coupled with, 3, 4
Self-injurious behavior
  biology of, 88–89
  dialectical behavior therapy and, 31
  hostile transferential feelings toward caregivers and, 118
  skills necessary to manage and prevent, 32–33
"Sequential pharmacodynamic interaction," 136–137
Serotonergic antidepressants, 133–134
Serotonin reuptake inhibitor antidepressants, 93, 138, 144–145
Sheeley v. Memorial Hospital, 156
Significant others. *See also* Family
  documenting comments and concerns of, 160
  as exterior sustaining resource, 192
  rehabilitation and engagement of, 125
Skills, application of, 32–33
Sobriety
  detaining patient until, for reliable assessment, 116–117
  perils of, 125–126
  reassessment during, 121
Social supports
  rehabilitation and engagement of, 125
  widening use of, 46
Somatic illness, as stressor in elderly suicides, 89
Specialized services, advocacy for coverage of, 201
Spokane Community Mental Health Center, Gatekeepers Program of, 96
Stabilization of suicidal substance abusers in managed care, 116–120
Standards for access to emergency care, 28

Standards of care, 154–156
  coordination of, 29
  national, 156, 162–163
Step-down program, 66–68, 82–83. *See also* Levels of care
Stop-loss insurance, 168
Stress, past responses to, 190
Stressors, 49, 62
Substance abuse, 111–129
  crisis assessment and presence of, 18
  dual diagnosis creep and, 68–70
  early identification of, 115
  pharmacotherapy for, 134–135
  suicidality and, 111–114
    alcohol abuse, 111, 112, 113
    other drugs, 113–114
  suicidal substance abusers in managed care, 114–126
    acute assessment and stabilization, 116–120
    adolescents, 60–61, 112
    clinical guidelines for working with, **127–128**
    follow-up care, 120, 122–124
    perils of sobriety, 125–126
    preventive care, 115
    reassessment, 121–122
    rehabilitation, 124–125
Suicidal ideation
  adolescent, 59–60
  pharmacotherapy and reduction of, 132–135
Suicidal intent, communication of, 93
Suicide attempts
  adolescent, 59, 112
  elderly, depression and, 91
  fantasies during, 61
  frequency of, 111–112
  precipitants to, 49
  by prescription drug overdose, 138–139
  self-induced illness from failed, 102
  by substance abusers, 112

Suicide completion
  common correlates of, 189–190
  managing aftermath of, 173–187
    affected groups, 174–177
    announcing what happened, 177, 180–181
    anticipatory component of treatment, 177, 178–180
    assessing meaning of suicide, 177, 184–185
    assisting affected groups in coping, 177, 181–184
  method chosen most frequently, 138
  substance abuse and, 112
Suicide crisis management. *See* Crisis care
Suicide prevention centers, 16
Suicide rate, 59–60, 77, 87
Supervision duties, 162–163
Sustaining resources, exterior, 192–193
Symptoms, determining potential seriousness of adolescent's, 82

Tabor v. Doctors Memorial Hospital, 161, 166
Tarasoff v. Regents of the University of California, 161
Team approach to care
  documentation in, 160
  during sobriety, 126
Teenagers. *See* Adolescents in managed care, suicidal
Tele-Help/Tele-Check service, 97
Telephone conversation, as immediate intervention, 19
Therapist. *See* Clinician(s)
Threats, using, 200
Tobacco use, suicide and, 112
Toxicology studies, 117

Trainees
  duty to supervise, 162–163
  mental health, standard of care for, 154
Training
  of personnel in crisis prevention centers, need for, 96
  workshop on depression and suicide in later life, 100
Transitional living facilities, 66
Transitions, preparing patients for, 83
Tranylcypromine, 135
Trauma survivors, 46
Triage in managed system, 41–44
Triage-oriented formulation, 44–48
Tricyclic antidepressants, 139, 144
Trifluoperazine, 134
Triggering stimulus, identifying possible, 46. *See also* Precipitants to suicide attempt
12-Step programs, 68

Undertreatment, 25–26, 144
Utilization management, 25, 26. *See also* Case management
Utilization manager, 23–24, 35, 166

Venlafaxine, 134
Vulnerability
  to despair, 190
  to life-threatening affects, 191–192

Warn, duty to, 161–162
Wickline v. State, 168, 201
Wilson v. Blue Cross of Southern California, 166, 200
Withholds, 167
Work, as exterior sustaining resource, 192–193